COURAGEOUS
CONFRONTATIONS

Cover design by Kim Johansen
Book design by Timm Bryson

All names, identifying characteristics, and other details
have been altered to protect patient privacy.

Library of Congress Cataloging-in-Publication Data

Helfant, Richard H.
Courageous confrontations : lives transformed by life-threatening illness / by Richard H. Helfant.-- 1st Sentient Publications ed.
p. cm.
ISBN 1-59181-035-3
1.   Critically ill--Psychology. 2.   Critically ill--Conduct of life. 3. Terminally ill--Psychology. 4.   Terminally ill--Conduct of life. I. Title.

R726.5.H44 2006
362.17'5--dc22

2005027118

Printed in the United States of America

10 9 8 7 6 5 4 3 2 1

SENTIENT PUBLICATIONS, LLC
1113 Spruce Street
Boulder, CO 80302
www.sentientpublications.com

Courageous Confrontations

Lives Transformed by Life-Threatening Illness

Richard H. Helfant, MD, FACC

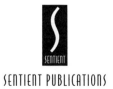

SENTIENT PUBLICATIONS

"At the bottom of the abyss comes the voice of salvation."

—Joseph Campbell

"Sweet are the uses of adversity."

—William Shakespeare

To my wife Barbara, whose love
blesses my life every day.
And to my miraculous grandchildren, Mia,
Benjamin, Elliott and David.

Contents

Acknowledgments

To my darling wife, Barbara, whose wisdom, sensitivity, and keen insights are reflected on every page—thank you with all my heart for accompanying me on this wonderful journey. Your deep love, unwavering support, and invaluable editing acumen helped to bring *Courageous Confrontations* into being.

My thanks as well to Steve, my multitalented son, whose sharp eye and editorial perceptiveness were vital contributions to the work. And to my wonderful daughter, Sharon, for her ongoing encouragement of the project.

I am most grateful to Jay Neugeboren, a mentor and compadre, for providing the indispensable gifts of his friendship and uniquely professional and personal perspectives. And my heartfelt thanks to two treasured colleagues, Lloyd Klein and Robert Katz, caring and compassionate physicians who added their sophistication, expertise, and medical input. I am deeply indebted as well to a lifelong friend, Judy Gelb, for bringing her discerning intelligence and judgment to the work.

In addition, I want to thank Phil Goldberg and James Stein for giving me astute advice and crucial feedback during the project's embryonic stages. Both were instrumental in helping me shape the themes of the book and give it cohesion.

Finally, I am indebted to my agent, Jodie Rhodes, for her remarkable dedication and commitment to the work and its author. And to Connie Shaw, an extraordinary publisher and person, for her thoughtfulness, friendship, and startling array of editing and publishing skills.

Introduction

"Wherever a thought goes, a chemical goes with it."
—Deepak Chopra, MD

Life-threatening illness is more than a crisis of the body; it is a crisis of the soul. During thirty-five years as a hospital-based cardiologist, I have seen innumerable ways in which patients react when faced with a medical catastrophe. Initially, most are overwhelmed, and feel as though they have been attacked by an alien force—as if body, mind, and spirit are under siege.

Many patients become paralyzed by fear. All resistance crumbles, replaced by passivity and resignation. Some go into denial, unwilling or unable to confront the enormity of what is happening. Yet others meet the crisis by challenging it head-on, and in the process, discover within themselves the resources to confront and overcome the gravest of circumstances. At times, these patients triumph, not because of the medical care they receive, but in spite of it.

There exists in all of us, a life force—the foundation of organic existence. In some, this drive is powerful and passionate. In others, there is ambivalence about continuing the burdensome business of living. When disease strikes, many are all too ready and even willing to have their lives end. But passivity or resignation are not immutable reactions to a life-threatening illness. My patients have taught me that the will to live can be awakened at any moment during its course.

Medical science has largely been blind to the power of a patient's mind in determining the outcome of an illness. Doctors are taught to view patients as the sum of their bodily parts, and to treat diseases by relying almost exclusively on the marvels of medical technology. Their unspoken communication to patients is unmistakable: We will mobilize our array of procedures and wonder drugs to save you. If they don't work, you are beyond help.

Having spent much of my career as an academic physician directing medical research programs, I have participated in the development of technological advances that have led to this new patient-care paradigm. While today's medical arsenal is invaluable in the combat against life-threatening illnesses, it has brought about a major side effect: far-reaching changes in the time-honored patient-doctor relationship.

That bond, once an invaluable component of the healing process, has become undermined. On teaching rounds, I have always felt it important to point out the ways in which doctors unwittingly discourage patients from mobilizing their inner resources to overcome an illness by implying that these elements play no part in the outcome. I emphasize how powerful these resources can be. Experience has taught me that they are comparable to any avant-garde pill or procedure.

This power was dramatically demonstrated to me many years ago by a patient named Vivian, who was suffering from progressive heart failure. The cumulative cardiac damage caused by several previous heart attacks had forced me to admit Vivian to the hospital three times in four months. Her heart had weakened to the point where it no longer responded to maximum doses of intravenous diuretics and other powerful medications. Edema fluid had accumulated in both her lungs and legs.

In the previous twenty-four hours, Vivian's kidneys had begun to shut down, making it impossible to treat the massive watery accumulations in her body. Her liver and other organ systems were also becoming affected. All therapeutic options had been exhausted. Vivian's chances for survival were close to zero.

After suffering for ten days in the intensive care unit, Vivian had had enough. "Look, Doctor," she said, "I am seventy-two years old. My husband has been dead for fifteen years, and my daughter hasn't spoken to me since the day he died. I'm in constant pain, and I have nothing to live for. Please let me go."

Despite their estrangement, Vivian had listed her daughter Janet as the person to be notified in the event of her death. When I asked whether Janet knew how sick she had been, Vivian shook her head.

"My daughter doesn't know, and I'm sure she doesn't care."

"If you wouldn't mind, I'd like to call her."

"I don't see the point. What good would it do?"

"It might not do any good, but I think your daughter should know what's going on with her mother."

"Frankly, I think it's a waste of time."

Two nights later, Janet came to the unit accompanied by her ten-year-old son, whom Vivian had never met.

The following morning, a different woman greeted me in the unit. Vivian looked at me, eyes glowing, and said, "My daughter is getting married in three weeks. She wants me to walk down the aisle with her." Tears welled up in Vivian's eyes as she took my hand and whispered, "I want to be there, Doctor."

Within days, Vivian's kidneys began to open up. The same dose of intravenous medication that had been ineffective now caused a substantial decrease in Vivian's edema fluid. After a week, her lungs were clear. By the end of week two, we were able to switch from intravenous to oral medications, and move Vivian out of the ICU.

Three days before discharge, Vivian began gingerly hobbling down the hospital corridor with the aid of a walker, the same one she used to walk down the aisle alongside Janet at her wedding.

Vivian not only attended her daughter's wedding, she also lived to attend her grandson's bar mitzvah three years later.

∞

Every doctor has seen patients with a life-threatening illness make a miraculous recovery after they were thought to be beyond hope. But because medical science is unable to explain these extraordinary occurrences, their importance is often ignored. Medicine is so enamored of the apparent infallibility of science that it has become blind to other possibilities. Remarkable recoveries like Vivian's are dismissed with the derisive term *anecdotal*, a code word for meaningless.

Countless times, I have observed two desperately ill patients lying side by side in the intensive care unit, seemingly in identical clinical circumstances. At the critical juncture, one would start to show signs of improvement and go on to live, while the other would go downhill, deteriorate, and die. The cause of that divergence has always been a profound mystery to me, and one of vital importance.

As a hospital-based cardiologist, I have repeatedly seen the importance of a patient's state of mind in determining the outcome of open-heart surgery. Most people, while admitting to feelings of anxiety and fear about having a heart operation, regard it as an unwelcome but necessary obstacle to overcome in order to proceed with their lives. Others become withdrawn, leaden with defeat, despite my repeated reassurances that their surgical risk was low and that all their studies indicated they would do well.

Often these patients did not do well. Sometimes they did not survive the operation. Once I became aware of this problem, or sensed that something was amiss, I began to visit with these patients before surgery.

One of my first conversations was with a woman named Claire, who was scheduled to have a heart valve repaired. When I asked how she felt about the operation, Claire's response was a noncommittal shrug.

"You don't think you're going to make it, do you?" I said.

At first startled, my patient nodded in agreement.

"Why?" I asked, "Everything is in your favor."

"My mother was only fifty-two years old when she died of a heart attack. She worked herself to death because she had to hold down a full-time job as a waitress, in order to raise me and my three brothers. I don't deserve to be here. I've already outlived her by six years."

Claire's story suggested that some patients, plagued by repressed guilt, convince themselves that death is imminent, and warranted as well. For the first time, I saw how important a patient's deep-seated beliefs and emotions can be in determining the outcome of an illness.

∞

Throughout history, physicians have understood that the mind has the power to harm as well as to heal. Recent research has now provided insights into how this comes about.

A heart attack is caused by the rupture of a cholesterol-laden deposit inside the wall of a coronary artery. A sudden surge in blood pressure, or spasm in a vulnerable artery, can erode its inner lining and result in a rupture. Circulating blood elements called platelets then adhere to the damaged artery surface, initiating a clot that occludes the vessel and causes a heart attack. But the core question remains. What *initiates* this lethal series of events?

Evidence has now made clear that mental stress increases blood pressure, constricts blood vessels, *and* increases the tendency of circulating platelets to form clots. When patients are stressed by performing difficult mental tasks in a laboratory setting, the identical circulatory responses can readily be elicited. Mental stress also causes sizeable deterioration in the cardiac function of patients with coronary artery disease.

It has become a cliché that depression is bad for our health, but only recently have its effects been scientifically studied. In a recent report, depression was shown to rival high cholesterol as a risk factor for coronary artery disease and heart attacks. Depression affects the circulation through mechanisms similar to those of stress.

Heart attacks usually occur during the early morning hours, when adrenalin and other stress hormones, as well as factors that cause clotting, are at peak activity. Surveys have found that 75 percent of working people dread getting up in the morning.

This dread is particularly intense on Monday mornings. The so-called "Monday morning blues" refers to a time when apprehension about having to confront the stresses of the long week ahead is at its peak. Most heart attacks occur on Monday.

While it has become generally accepted that our state of mind plays some role in health and disease, most people believe that the ultimate determinant of longevity resides in their genes. Whenever I have asked a patient how long he or she expects to live, their first instinct is to say,

"Well, my mother died at age X, and my father... ." This is another way of saying that my genes are my fate.

The twenty-first century has been heralded as the age of the genome, and medical genetics is widely touted as the future of health care. Diseases will soon be diagnosed by identifying the faulty gene; therapy will either fix or replace it. While genes are an undeniably important factor in causing disease, their role has been vastly overemphasized. For the most common diseases, such as cancer and atherosclerosis, genes are predispositions—*not* inevitabilities.

Identical twins have the same genetic risk for disease, yet several studies have shown substantial differences in their health histories. This is because of another crucial factor in determining one's propensity for disease: an individual's environment. According to Craig Venter, former CEO of the company that first decoded the human genome, "The wonderful diversity of the human species is not hard-wired in our genetic code. Our environments are critical."

A recent report in *The New England Journal of Medicine* studied 44,788 twins to evaluate the comparative importance of genes and the environment in causing the most common types of cancer. The study concluded: "Inherited genetic factors make a minor contribution to susceptibility in most types of cancer. The overwhelming contributor to the causation of cancer is the environment." It is now widely accepted that 80 to 90 percent of human cancer is due to nongenetic factors.

The overriding importance of environmental elements is also clear in the development of atherosclerosis, the number one killer in the United States. Atherosclerosis is a multifactorial disorder resulting from an interaction of several predisposing abnormalities such as high cholesterol, hypertension, and diabetes. Research has conclusively shown that reducing these risks substantially decreases the probability of having a heart attack or stroke. For example, a loss of just 7 percent of body weight in obese people reduces the incidence of diabetes by 58 percent, while shedding ten pounds will normalize the blood pressure of those with borderline hypertension, no matter what their genetic propensity.

The human genome project has given us a more nuanced under-standing of how genes work. It is now clear that they are not static blue-prints that dictate our biological behavior. Most genes have switches, called *promoters*, that control how, when, and even *if* they become active—a phenomenon known as gene *expression*. Other regulatory ele-ments, called gene *enhancers*, also play a role. Even slight alterations in promoters or enhancers can lead to dramatic changes in gene expression. But the factors that determine whether or not genes are turned on or off, and for how long, remain largely unknown.

Animal studies have begun to show that social, behavioral, and envi-ronmental elements can determine whether or not genes are expressed. For example, stress has been demonstrated to cause diabetes in genetical-ly prone animals, while those with the same genetic susceptibilities that are not exposed to stress are less likely to develop the disease.

Recent insights into Pavlov's famous conditioning experiments in dogs provide another striking example. A century ago, the Russian scien-tist showed that the brain of dogs could be trained to anticipate the arrival of food. We now know that this type of training changes the brain through the expression of seventeen genes that have been given the name CREB genes.

These findings demonstrate that a change in mental conditioning not only affects gene expression, but also can actually change the way our genes operate. They prove that our genes no longer should be thought of as immutable determinants of our fate, but as dynamic entities, switching on and off in response to outside influences, as much the result as the cause of our mental, emotional, and biological processes.

∞

Genetic diseases generally fall into one of three categories. The first, called chromosomal disorders, are caused either by an excess or a deficient number of genes. Down's syndrome is an example of this type of disorder. The second, referred to as simple inherited disorders, are primarily deter-mined by a single abnormally altered or mutant gene. An example is sick-le cell anemia, a disease affecting red blood cells.

The last and most common group is called multifactorial disorders, because they result from an interaction of multiple genetic and environmental factors. Coronary artery disease and most cancers fall into this category. Genetics experts agree that the risk of inheriting a disease is substantially lower in the multifactor group than it is in the first two groups.

Experience has convinced me that in addition to genes themselves, our minds' conclusions about our genes—something I call *mental genetics*—also has a major influence on our health and longevity. When we conclude that our parents' medical histories and their life spans determine our own, that belief can create its own reality.

People with a strong will to live understand that when they take life-enhancing measures, their health and longevity will be favorably affected regardless of their genes. They take responsibility for their lives instead of being victims of events.

∞

Of the innumerable patients I have seen over my medical lifetime, those in this book have remained alive in my memory because of their vivid, larger-than-life personalities, courage, and remarkable responses to medical crises. *Courageous Confrontations* tells their stories.

Initially, several of them could not acknowledge the massive disruption to their compulsive, driven lives. But ultimately, each patient discovered an untapped source of inner strength that imposed new realities on his or her illness, and each emerged from the crisis with an awakened spiritual dimension. Viewing their former selves from a heightened perspective, most rejected the goals of the past. As old truths shattered and new landscapes formed, they began to live in accord with deeper ranges of their existential essence. Several found fulfillment by devoting themselves to healing others or the planet.

∞

Emily Dickinson wrote: "We never know how tall we can be until we are called on to rise." All of us have the capacity to grow, transform, and enrich the quality of our lives as well as the lives of others. It is my hope that the stories in this book will inspire you, the reader, to similar awakenings.

The Mafia Kingpin

"Thou best of thieves, who with an easy key dost steal us from ourselves."
—John Dryden

T here's a patient sitting in my office about to have a coronary," Tony whispered over the phone. "The guy is one of the most powerful people in New York. He could shut down the city with a phone call, but the stresses he's under are unreal. The man deals with maybe fifteen crises a day, and he's got the blood pressure to prove it. I keep telling him to slow down, but he won't listen. You know the type. I'm sure you have a car-load of VIP patients just like him."

"Make that a truckload," I said with a chuckle.

Tony Vincent and I went back a long way. We had been classmates and good friends at NYU-Bellevue Medical School. Most of our fellow students were nerdy workaholics, well suited to the medical school grind, but Tony was different. He had style and panache, and knew how to have a good time. Somehow, Tony always managed to have complimentary front row tickets for all the prime time events. Together we saw the biggest ball games, boxing matches, and rock concerts at Madison Square Garden and Yankee Stadium. But years had past since I last heard from him.

"Al's been a chain-smoker all his life," Tony continued. "And the way he eats! Whenever I try getting him to cut down, he just laughs at me. I don't have to tell you how we Italians love our food. Remember the old days?"

"I sure do. Those were great times."

∞

Tony had frequently invited me to his parents' Long Island estate for their Friday night dinner parties. After a week of dissecting formaldehyde-soaked cadavers and getting bleary-eyed squinting through microscopes, I always looked forward to the extravaganzas. I could still see the preening men in long cashmere overcoats and wide-brimmed fedoras, smoking foul-smelling cigars, making their regal entrances, trailed by dutiful wives fussing over litters of children.

Everyone gorged lustily on the sumptuous meals, which included soup, antipasto, and endless platters of pasta and meats, and which were lubricated with copious quantities of whisky and red wine. Tony's father, a general practitioner, loved to engage with his guests in banter that played on the word *health*. Amid raucous laughter, the sinister-sounding language often was punctuated by animated discussions about the health of a business or the health of friends and associates. These larger-than-life characters mesmerized me, but whenever I asked Tony about them, he waved away my questions.

After completing his training, Tony astounded everyone by passing up an opportunity to join a lucrative medical group practice on Park Avenue. Instead, he joined his father in Brooklyn.

"Anyway," Tony said, "the point is, my patient's been having chest pains on and off for several months. I've been after him to see a cardiologist, but he never took it seriously. Lately it's gotten worse, and today he looks terrible. For the past two weeks, he's been getting the pains after walking just half a block. Now it's gotten so bad, he's stopped walking altogether. Dick, for pain to stop this man, it's got to be pretty damn severe. Last night, it hit him at home while he was watching TV."

The symptoms Tony described had all the earmarks of angina pectoris, the chest pains that occur when the cholesterol deposits in the wall of one or more of the coronary arteries supplying blood and oxygen to the heart become so advanced that they cause a partial obstruction of blood flow to the cardiac muscle.

When a patient with a severe coronary obstruction engages in physical activity, the heart muscle requires more blood and oxygen than the blocked artery can deliver. The symptoms that result are usually experienced as pressure sensations that feel like constricting, suffocating, or squeezing in the center of the chest, although they may also occur in the shoulders (more frequently the left), arms, neck, or jaw.

The word *angina* comes from the Greek, meaning "strangling." References to it can be found in ancient Egyptian and Greek writings, and even in the Bible. In 1772, the first detailed description of the symptoms was written by William Heberden, an English physician. It has never been surpassed. "There is a disorder of the breast marked with strong and peculiar symptoms, and one who is afflicted with it is seized while walking with a painful and most disagreeable symptom which seems as if it would extinguish life if it were to continue. But the moment one stands still, all this unpleasantness vanishes."

While the presence of angina is disquieting evidence of advanced coronary artery disease, any change in the pattern of a patient's symptoms signals imminent danger. An increase in the frequency or severity of the chest pain indicates that the coronary obstructions are no longer stable. It suggests that one of them may have ruptured, leaving it defenseless against blood elements called platelets that lead to the formation of a clot (a thrombus). When a thrombus occludes a coronary artery, the result is a heart attack (a coronary thrombosis).

Tony's patient had experienced a distinct change in the pattern of his anginal chest pains. Most worrisome was the episode while watching TV, because his heart was at rest. Patients who have anginal symptoms while sedentary are at the highest risk.

Tony was right about his friend being in jeopardy. The man could have a life-threatening heart attack at any time.

∞

"Sounds serious," I said. "You better get your patient to a cardiologist as soon as possible."

"I want you to see him."

"Tony, I'm in Philadelphia, and you're in Brooklyn. Your patient is too sick and too unstable to come all the way down here. He could have a coronary on the way. You need to hospitalize him immediately. I'm sure you know plenty of first-rate cardiologists in New York. If not, I can..."

"Listen to me, my friend. I have a big problem here, and I need your help. Al is family. He's one of my father's closest friends. They grew up together. The man is a second father to me. You understand?"

"Sure, but I still think..."

"You are not listening! It's already been decided. You are the guy." Tony lowered his voice and continued. "I know this may sound strange, but trust is indispensable to my friend. He likes that you and I are old friends, that we went to school together, and that you knew my family from the old days. Besides, he wants to take care of this out of town. Al doesn't want his business associates to know he's sick."

Finally I gave in, agreeing to see Tony's friend in my office at one o'clock the following afternoon.

At eleven-thirty the next morning, I was completing rounds when my secretary Jean burst into the coronary care unit. "I need to see you!" she shouted.

"What's going on?" I said, after rushing her to a quiet corner.

"Two of the creepiest men I ever saw are in the office looking for you. They just marched in like they owned the place, and when I asked what they wanted, one of them said he had an appointment. I looked at the list of today's office patients and saw that no new people were scheduled. When I started to explain that he didn't have an appointment and would have to leave, the guy leans over my desk, gets right in my face, and tells me he's staying until he sees you. Then he pulls out this huge roll of hundred dollar bills, peels one off, hands it to me, and says, 'Look, Doll. You take this, and go tell the doc Tony's friend is here.' Do you know someone named Tony?"

"Doll? Jesus..."

"So I say, 'I don't want your money, and if you don't leave, I'll have to call hospital security.' Well, he turns scarlet, rises up like King Kong, and snarls, 'Look, Doll, if you don't get the doc over here, I'll go find him myself.'"

Jean must be exaggerating, I thought. Smiling tightly, I said, "Rounds are just about over. Go back to the office and tell him politely that I'll be there in a few minutes."

An incredulous look came over Jean's face. "What are you saying? Do you *know* this person?"

∞

After rounds, I adjusted my lab coat, took a deep breath, and headed for the office. Outside the suite, a squat man with the massive arms and belly of a sumo wrestler, and a toupee that looked like a small animal rescued from an oil spill, paced back and forth across the hall. When he turned toward me, I managed a smile and stuck out my hand.

"Not me," he said, staring at my outstretched hand as if it were covered with fungus. "He's over there."

Together, we walked into the patient waiting area. There, sitting alone, a vast, gray-haired man, dressed like the CEO of a Fortune 500 company in a dark, double-breasted silk suit, a white dress shirt adorned with gold and diamond-studded cufflinks, and black alligator loafers, sat reading a copy of *The Wall Street Journal*.

When he saw us, a sneer passing for a smile slowly spread across his fleshy lips, revealing decayed, cigarette-stained teeth. As he slowly uncoiled from the chair, his steel-gray eyes, deeply set above a huge hooked nose, stared straight into mine. He exuded a primal energy, like a sated lion that had just hunted down and devoured its prey.

As the man moved slowly toward me, he continued to grin, while his eyes continued their interrogation.

I mumbled, "Nice to meet you, Mr....."

"Al," the surprisingly high, thin voice said. "Just call me Al."

∞

This was my old medical school buddy's family friend. The big-time businessman who rubs elbows with the New York movers and shakers. Mr. Mogul, who could shut down the city with a phone call. The man looked more like the king of the jungle than the king of New York.

I was furious with Tony, but there seemed no choice but to go ahead. Telling myself to stay calm, to be "the doctor," I led Al into an exam room, his pit bull trailing closely behind. Turning to him, I said, "It might be better if Al and I did this alone."

"I go with Big Al. I always go with Big Al."

Big Al! My god, I thought to myself. No wonder Tony had conveniently neglected to tell me his patient's name.

"Hey, Freddie, show the doc here some respect." Each word was like a fist forcing its way through clenched, decaying teeth.

"I thought you might want to tell me some things in private," I said, struggling to maintain what was left of my composure.

"That's okay, Doc, I can tell you anything in front of my friend here. Right Freddo?" The pit bull nodded deferentially.

After Big Al confirmed the nature of his chest pain symptoms, it was time for the physical examination.

"Al," I said, handing him a paper gown while reaching for an air of casual authority, "you'll need to remove your clothes and put this on for the physical exam."

Big Al abruptly stopped unbuttoning his suit jacket. "Hey Doc, it's only the ticker that's the problem, knowwhatImean?"

I explained that it was important to do a complete physical.

"No problem," he replied evenly. His boxer shorts, shoes, and socks stayed on.

During a physical exam, most patients become passive and listless. Frequently, their eyes close or they stare into space. But as I took Big Al's massive hand and began probing for a pulse, his eyes remained fixed on me, scrutinizing every movement. I felt as though *I* were the one being evaluated.

Al reeked like an ashtray filled with yesterday's cigarette butts. Years of heavy smoking had seriously impaired his breathing, and even the minor exertion of getting on the exam table left him wheezing like a cogwheel train puffing up a steep hill. Because of his shortness of breath, Big Al had to purse his lips simply to exhale.

I studied his fingernails, noting the bluish-purple discoloration that indicated inadequate oxygen supply, due to a sluggish circulation caused by his heart disease, or lung damage from the smoking, or both. As Tony had warned, Big Al's blood pressure was sky high. A reading of 135 over 85 is the upper range of normal. Big Al's pressure was 155 over 98.

When I listened to his lungs, loud wheezes and whistling noises roared into my ears. The distorted breathing pattern was evidence of severe emphysema, the most common pulmonary abnormality caused by cigarette smoking.

Placing my right hand over Big Al's fleshy left breast, I felt his heart. It was abnormally enlarged either because of the high blood pressure or a previous heart attack. In any case, it was clear from the physical that Big Al had both severe heart and lung disease.

Big Al's electrocardiogram revealed further evidence of his tenuous and alarming condition. It showed abnormalities called pathologic Q waves. Q waves are the hallmarks of cardiac damage caused by a previous heart attack. Abnormalities were also present on another portion of the EKG called the ST segment. The segment was deeply depressed all across his chest, yet another harbinger of impending danger. While Big Al dressed, I told him about my concern.

"Al, I'm afraid Tony was right. You have a serious problem. There's a real risk that you could have a massive heart attack at any time. I'd like to admit you to the hospital immediately, so we can take care of you before anything happens."

Seemingly oblivious to what I was saying, Big Al scrutinized himself in the mirror, meticulously combing his hair.

"We need to get special x-rays called angiograms. They are pictures of your coronary arteries—the blood vessels going to your heart. The test is done in a specialized procedure room called a catheterization laboratory. We insert a catheter, a long, thin plastic tube in one of your groin vessels, thread it up to your heart, send dye through it, and take the x-ray pictures. If they show that your arteries are badly blocked, I'll probably have to recommend a heart operation, called a coronary bypass. In your case, the risk is going to be quite…"

Before I could go any further, Big Al turned toward me, flashed a tooth-stained grin, and held up a hand. Settling into a nearby chair, he stretched out his arms and legs in an open-body position and motioned me to sit beside him. The man seemed as calm as a balloon floating across a clear blue sky.

"Tony tells me you were good pals in school. Regular *paisans*. I like that. Tony's a good boy. His father's been doctoring me and mine thirty, forty years. We're close, like family, knowwhatImean? You're from Brooklyn too, right Doc? What part of Brooklyn did you grow up in? I bet it was Flatbush."

To my amazement, Big Al seemed intent on ignoring everything I told him about my plan to get him through his life-threatening medical condition. Why? At a time like this, what in the world did Brooklyn have to do with anything?

"Bet all your pals were smart Jewish kids, studying all the time so they could become rich doctors or blood-sucking lawyers, right?" Big Al turned to Freddie with a smirk. "Nothing like us. All we had was trouble. Tell the doc, Freddo?"

On cue, Freddie began to speak, his voice filled with reverence and passion. "In our neighborhood, Big Al's like the Pope. Everybody loves him." He lowered his voice. "Big Al is a great man."

Pleased by the pit bull's flattery, Big Al continued. "My neighborhood was nothing like yours. The streets where I grew up were tough. Am I right, Freddo?"

The pit bull nodded.

"I never made it past eighth grade. I was a butcher's kid—a nothing. While you were studying in school, I was carving and packing sides of beef. Always covered with blood and guts. I was at the shop five o'clock every morning. Pitch black outside. Everybody else in the whole world still asleep." Big Al held up his huge hands. "See these? Handled enough meat to feed all of New York before I was fifteen.

"But by the time I was nineteen, I was wearing suits with the big lapels and imported silk ties with solid gold collar pins pushing the Windsor up nice and smart."

"And the handmade Italian shoes," the pit bull chimed in.

"You were still a snot nose kid and I was already making real money, looking fine," Al continued. "While you were learning books, I was learning the streets, who's who and what's what. KnowwhatImean?

"You and me, we've both come a long way. Look at you. Big, famous heart doctor. And me, a self-made American businessman. Dignified. Respected. I've got beautiful tailor-made suits, cashmere coats, my own table at the best restaurants in New York. Dining and socializing with the heads of corporations, heads of the unions, politicians. Name it. I know everybody. Two boys from Brooklyn made it to the big-time. We did pretty good, knowwhatImean?"

There was a knock on the exam room door. When I asked who it was, my office nurse peeked in, rolled her eyes, and gave me her best "we're-drowning-in-patients-and-I've-run-out-of-excuses" look. Furtively, I glanced at my watch. Big Al's reminiscences had been fascinating, but he still seemed oblivious to his surroundings and his dire medical situation.

"Al," I said, resuming my physician's tone, "we really need to talk about your problem."

Big Al put up a hand to silence me. "When you were a kid in Brooklyn, you were nothing. Now, you are a very important, big-shot doctor, too busy to talk about anything but fancy x-rays and heart operations."

Then, flashing a grin and shifting gears, he said, "Hey Doc, Tony said you're of the Jewish faith. That right?"

"Yes," I said warily, half-wondering where he was going now, but determined to end this and get back to my other patients. "Al, we just have to…"

Big Al would not hear anything he did not want to hear. He went on as if I had not uttered a word.

"That's good. I like Jews. We always got along with the Jews, right, Freddo? They had to make it on their own when they came over here, same as us. Not like the people who own this country and set everything up just for themselves. They made all the rules, and put all the legal bull-shit together so they got the power to keep the Italians and the Jews under their thumb. You're okay, Doc. I'll come into your hospital. You do your fancy x-ray, and let me know what's what."

"I won't be doing the test myself tomorrow, Al. My schedule…"

Big Al stuck a finger into my face. "You're doing that test on me, Doc. Only you. Tomorrow. That's what Tony said. You."

"Al, there are several other specialists on our staff who are more qual-ified to do the test than I am."

Leaning in closer, Big Al grabbed my forearm. "You," he whispered like an ill wind, straight into my ear. "Just you, Doc."

"Okay. If that's what Tony promised, I'll do your angiogram."

Slowly, Big Al released me. "You're okay, Doc. Just like Tony said. Nice Jewish kid from Brooklyn. Flatbush. I like you. Okay, it's decided. Tomorrow."

∞

The coronary angiogram, done the following morning, showed that all three of Big Al's major coronary arteries were more than 90 percent blocked. In addition, as the physical exam and electrocardiogram suggest-ed, a large portion of his cardiac muscle was damaged from a previous heart attack.

The best indicator of overall heart function is a measurement called the ejection fraction, the fraction of blood that is ejected from the heart with each beat. Normally, the ejection fraction is 50 percent or more. Big Al's ejection fraction was only 35 percent. The low number added a con-siderable risk to his bypass operation.

Before talking to Big Al about the test results, I met my medical rounding team in the radiology department. Since Al's abnormal lungs made him susceptible to pulmonary complications after anesthesia, I needed to evaluate his chest x-ray.

∞

As we gathered in a semicircle around the x-ray viewer, it was immedi-ately apparent that Big Al's heart was enlarged and that severe emphyse-ma had seriously distorted his lungs. Then, something else caught my eye.

Quickly making the connection, I kept my composure long enough to provide a little teaching lesson on how to interpret an unusual x-ray.

"Phillip," I said to the medical student who had been assigned to Big Al, "tell us what you see in this patient's x-ray."

"Well, the heart's enlarged, and lungs are…uh, I'm not sure…"

"Those Kerley B lines indicate heart failure, don't you think?" I said, helping him along. Phillip nodded absently. Kerley B lines are wavy densities on a chest x-ray that reflect fluid collections in the lungs resulting from heart failure.

"How about the severe hyperinflation of the lungs caused by our patient's heavy smoking? Pretty bad emphysema, don't you think?"

Turning to one of the interns, I moved to the abnormality that had surprised me. "Jim, tell us what you think about the right clavicle. See anything unusual?"

"Something's there, but I don't know what it is."

"Just describe it," I said. "What's its shape?"

"Looks like a tapered cylinder, blunt on the end," Joan, one of our bright residents said. "Kind of metallic, like…"

"Geez," Phillip blurted out, "that thing looks like a bullet—lodged in the guy's collarbone!"

∞

Sitting up in bed, Big Al scrutinized the retinue entering his room. "What's all this?" he said, looking at me. "What am I, a freak show in some fuckin' circus? I told you before Doc, I just want you."

"It's okay, Al. These young doctors are just helping. I'm in charge."

"Yeah? What kind of help do you need?" Reluctantly, he leaned back, allowing me to proceed.

"We just looked at your chest x-ray, and there's a bullet in your right collarbone."

"What about it?"

"It's important that we know how long it's been there, and if it's bothered you in any way."

"It doesn't bother me."

"When did you get it?" I asked.

Big Al paused. "In the war."

Behind me, one of the students said in a loud whisper, "Right. The war on South Street."

Amid hushed chuckles, Big Al bolted upright, eyes flaring and bellowed, "Who the fuck said that? You snot-nosed little bastards don't think I did my duty for this country against Mussolini and Hitler?" Suddenly, he grabbed his chest and grimaced in pain.

"Easy Al," I pleaded, while shaking my head at the medical student. "He didn't mean anything."

Big Al fell back on his pillow. "Dumb sumbitch. None of you knows shit. All the things we did for the government. They begged us." Rising up, he roared at the stunned students. "All you snot noses—get out. Now!"

Waving the group out of the room, my focus stayed on Big Al. My patient was still clutching his chest, and he needed medication to relieve it.

"Al," I said softly, "You need nitroglycerin for the pain. I'll run over to the nurses' station and be right back."

"You're not going anywhere, Doc. You're going to stay right here and listen." Big Al took a deep breath, and looked at me steadily. I could see that the chest pain was easing.

"You grew up in Brooklyn, but you don't know shit about the docks. Nobody knows what went on down there during the war. Those Nazi bastards were doing all this sabotage. All kinds of shit was going on. They blew up our ships and the government lied like they always do, so people wouldn't get scared. The newspapers were saying this ship or that ship got blown up by accident. Bullshit. The government came crawling on their hands and knees, begging us to take care of the Nazis. Fucking Germans were disrupting all the shipping down there.

"And guess what? The word came down, and we took care of it. Let me tell you something. Those Nazi bastards were tough! But we were tougher."

Big Al sighed and leaned back on his pillow. "Want to know what thanks we got? Shit, that's what. You ask Tony sometime. He knows the story. Then you tell your little snot noses who saved their country's ass. You tell them."

"I will, Al."

When Big Al's chest pain abated and he seemed sufficiently relaxed, I began to tell him about the angiogram and the heart surgery.

"Al, I'm afraid you're going to need…"

Big Al raised a hand. "Yeah, I know. The ticker is fucked up and I need the operation, right?" I nodded.

"Okay, Doc, you set it up." Then he said, "Two things. You stay with me the whole time of the operation. No snot noses. Just you. The whole time. And Freddie, he stays too. I want you and Freddie there the whole time they got me out with the gas."

"Be reasonable, Al. Freddie can't go into the operating room. It would cause…"

Once again, the hand went out. "I already told you, Doc. Freddie goes where I go. Freddie stays where I stay. Wherever. Right, Freddo?"

"Goddamn right," the pit bull muttered.

I knew better than to argue. "As long as Freddie promises to stay in a corner of the operating room so he doesn't get in the way. I'll tell the staff he's a visiting doctor, or something."

"Yeah. My man Freddo, the visiting doctor from Sicily," Big Al said, roaring at his own joke. "Hey Doc. Don't you worry about Freddie. He'll be quiet like a church mouse. Right, Freddo?

"One more thing. I'm not worried about the pain. I can handle pain. But I don't like that tube Tony told me about. The thing they put down my throat for the gas. I want it out as soon as the operation's over. I told Tony, and he said talk to you."

"I understand how you feel, Al, but your lungs are in very bad shape because of all the cigarette smoking. The anesthetic, the gas that puts you under during the operation, can cause an inflammation in the lungs. In heavy smokers like you, we usually have to wait until the morning after surgery before it's safe to remove the tube."

"Doc, you are not listening again. I want that thing out right after the operation."

∞

Relieved that the day was over, I drove home that evening, entered the house, and as usual dropped to my knees anticipating that the kids would race out for their customary bear hugs. Sharon squealed her usual "Daddy's home," but Stevie had a quiet glint in his eye, as if he had just spotted the Cookie Monster materialize from under his bed.

"You got three calls, Dad," he said. "I wrote them all down." Squinting to decipher his scribbles, Stevie continued, "Johnny from Boston, Sal from New York, and Frankie from Chicago. They wanted to know about somebody called Big Al. Who's Big Al?"

"He's a patient in the hospital," I said, hiding my shock. "What did they want?"

"Those guys sounded really weird. Dropping his chin to his chest, Stevie feigned a deep voice. They said stuff like, 'This is Johnny from Boston. Tell the doc I want to talk to him about Big Al.' Something like that. Then they gave me their phone numbers."

I reflexively stood bolt upright, the shocked look on my face immediately apparent.

"Is something wrong, Dad?" Sharon said.

"No...no...nothing's wrong. Thanks, Stevie. You've been a big help, as always. I'll call them back, and after that we can have some fun, okay?"

Who were these people? What did they want? And how did they get my unlisted home phone number? Taking a deep breath, I went into my study and dialed the first number.

"This Big Al's doc?"

"Yes. How can I help you?"

"You're gonna take good care of Big Al, right Doc? You need to take real good care of him. We're close, me and Al. Real close. Grew up together. Let me ask you something, Doc. You sure he really needs this operation?"

"Yes, I am."

"I hope you're right, Doc. I sure hope you're right. Big Al's gonna make it through this operation, ain't he, Doc?"

"Well, I think so, but there are several things that are not in his favor. He has a lot of heart damage, and his cigarette smoking has..."

"You get Big Al through the operation, Doc. You're supposed to be the best. Just get him through." There was a click, followed by dial tone.

Staring at the phone, I tried to reassure myself that this frightening intrusion into my home would disappear once Big Al survived the surgery and returned to New York. All I had to do was get him through safely and all would be well. The phone began to ring again, but I decided to ignore it, and it soon stopped. I was about to leave the study when Stevie burst in.

"Dad, it's Vinnie from Las Vegas. He wants to talk to you about that Big Al guy. Boy, your patient must really be famous."

The calls continued throughout the night.

∞

Prior to surgery the following morning, I went to see Big Al. I normally do this to assess my patient's state of mind and to reassure them that everything possible would be done to get them safely through the operation. But today, it felt like the situation was reversed. After those not-so-veiled threats by Big Al's phone friends, *I* needed as much reassurance as my patient.

When he saw me, a knowing smile came over Big Al's face. "Hey Doc, I hear you got a couple calls last night."

"As a matter of fact, I did."

"Make you nervous, Doc? Well, don't worry. I'm going to do just fine. Remember when Freddo told you about my neighborhood in Brooklyn?"

"Sure."

"Well, those people depend on me, and there's no way I'm letting them down. Those Long Island punks are just waiting to step in and take over everything, but I swear to Christ, I'm not going anywhere. KnowwhatImean?"

Big Al stared into my eyes, a fierce resolve exuding from every pore of his being. I had spent a sleepless night tortured by possibilities of disaster—everything from the seepage of air into Big Al's bloodline, or the slip of a gloved hand at a critical surgical moment, to an idiosyncratic reaction of his body to the general anesthesia or a host of other medications. Then there was what I called the final moment of truth—that always uncertain time when a patient had to come off the heart bypass machine—the moment when his heart would once again be called on to beat on its own. As I met Big Al's eyes, all of my fears evaporated.

"I sure do," I said.

∞

The operation did go well. When it was completed, I left the surgical suite to check on some patients. It would be at least an hour before Big Al woke up from the anesthesia and was transferred to the surgical intensive care unit.

Before reaching my first patient, I heard my name being paged. Helene, the surgical unit head nurse, came on the line.

"What's up?" I asked.

"Get over here fast! Your patient, the one who just came out of the operating room, just extubated himself, and he's in trouble. The man's going crazy. He's coughing his lungs out, and he's about to become asphyxiated."

"You mean he pulled out the breathing tube by himself?" I screamed into the phone. "He shouldn't even be awake yet. Call Anesthesia. Tell them to get somebody over to the unit, and get that damned tube back in. I'll be right there."

"We already called, and they're sending someone. But your patient won't let anybody near him, and he's deteriorating fast…turning gray and…"

"I'm on my way."

As I entered the unit, a surreal scene confronted me. Propped up on both elbows, and looking like an ashen apparition, Big Al sat enmeshed in a tangle of disconnected intravenous tubes, catheters, and monitor wires, violently coughing up gobs of foul sputum, and vowing to kill anybody who came near. A cadre of cowering doctors and nurses stood several feet from the foot of his bed, begging for permission to save him by replacing the breathing tube and restoring the lines.

As I approached, Big Al's coughing spasm began to subside. "Anybody comes near me dies. Where is my doc? I told him, no fuckin' tube."

"I'm right here, Al." Determined to appear calm, I quietly moved everyone back, trusting that my medical instincts would somehow allow me to get control of the situation. "What's going on, Al?"

"What does it fuckin' look like?" Big Al said, panting for breath. "You keep them away." Another coughing spasm began, with thick wads of sputum spraying over the sheets.

Blotting out the chaos, I focused on two things: making a careful assessment of my patient's clinical situation, and regaining his trust.

"Al," I said softly, "I promise, nobody will do anything to you unless…"

"No fuckin' tube." Big Al leaned back and stared at the ceiling, gasping for breath.

When I nodded in seeming agreement, Big Al's breathing slowed. In all my years of caring for patients after open-heart surgery, I had never seen anything like this. How could anyone be fully awake so soon after general anesthesia? After clearing that last great gob of sputum, some color had returned to his face, and his respirations deepened and slowed. Those were good signs. In evaluating a patient's pulmonary function, the depth and frequency of his respirations are critical indicators. In Big Al's case, they suggested that perhaps his lungs might be able to do the job of delivering life-giving oxygen to his fragile, vulnerable heart without the respirator.

The anesthesiologist who had been called to replace the tube had already arrived and stood behind me. Tapping me on the shoulder, he whispered, "This is an emergency. If we don't get him tubed…"

"I know," I whispered back, watching while Al continued to stare at the ceiling. "But look how awake he is. And his breathing pattern looks pretty normal now. Slow and deep. Maybe if he has already coughed up all that gunk… just maybe we can get away without…"

"You've got to be kidding! I'm telling you right now, there is no way this guy can survive without being tubed."

"I hear you, but let's not panic. Why don't we check and see how much he really needs the tube? It'll only take a minute or two. We can run some quick blood gas tests and get a portable chest x-ray. If they're okay, and his respirations stay normal, we just might be able to get away with putting him on a high-flow oxygen mask. I'm going to have a listen to his lungs. Hang in there with me."

Approaching Big Al, I took out my stethoscope. "Al, I want to examine your heart and lungs, and have one of the nurses take some blood from your arm. It will help us to see how you're doing. Okay?"

Sitting upright, Big Al met my eyes. The ghastly gray look was gone, and his respirations continued slow and deep.

"Just you and her." Coughing briefly, he moved back onto his pillows, while monitoring my every move.

I asked Big Al to inhale deeply, while I listened to his lungs. Air was coursing throughout all of his lung fields. I smiled reassuringly at my patient, patted him on the shoulder, and walked back to the group.

"It's amazing. His respirations are normal."

"For now," the anesthesiologist said. "But he could easily become fatigued, and if he does, the respirations will become too shallow. What then?"

To my relief, the portable x-ray confirmed that all portions of Big Al's lungs were receiving air normally. The blood gas study showed that an adequate amount of oxygen was getting into his system.

"Let's put him on the high-flow oxygen mask," I said. "Get serial blood studies for the next several hours, and monitor his respirations every fifteen minutes. Any deterioration and I'll try like hell to talk him into having the tube reinserted. Okay?"

"You are out of your mind," the anesthesiologist said. "*I'm* having nothing to do with this."

At a little past nine that night, I made my last visit to the unit before going home. To everyone's amazement, Big Al continued to do remarkably well. He had not gotten fatigued, his respirations had remained deep, and his breathing rate was stable. He was on the oxygen mask, and the blood studies stayed normal. All evidence now pointed to a rapid recovery.

The unit was quiet. Visiting hours had just ended, and most of the patients were asleep. In the distance, an intern whispered to a nurse. The rest of the doctors had gone for the day. A handful of nurses went about their chores as I approached his bed. Big Al was asleep. The ever-vigilant Freddie sat unobtrusively in a corner. Gently, I placed my stethoscope at the base of Big Al's chest.

Suddenly, a figure wearing a camel hair coat, with thick, tinted eyeglasses on a cherubic face, appeared at the foot of the bed. As Freddie began to rise from his chair, the man turned and gestured at him to sit back down. The goon hesitated, then obeyed. Turning to face me, the man put his hand on my arm. Wordlessly, he nodded at Big Al. The message was clear: *Go about your business, and get lost. Forget you ever laid eyes on me.*

Without waking Big Al, I concluded my examination and checked his lab test results. Everything was in order. Silently, I backed away, and left the unit for the refuge of home.

As I was heading for the doctors' parking lot through the hospital lobby, a newspaper stand carrying the evening edition of *The Philadelphia Inquirer* caught my eye. A boldface headline read—NATIONWIDE FBI MANHUNT FOR ANGELO BRUNO, MAFIA DON OF PHILADELPHIA. Below was a large picture of a cherubic-faced man with thick, tinted eyeglasses. It was the man I had seen in the unit moments before.

∞

For the next two days, everything stayed on course. Al was in great spirits. After his move out of the unit into a private suite, the nurses and hospital administrators ignored the flagrant violations of their visiting rules, as a strange assortment of characters began to wander in and out at all hours.

On the third night, a group of Big Al's friends joined him to celebrate his recovery. They lit up cigarettes and cigars, and toasted him with champagne. When Mandy, the night-duty nurse, entered the room to give Al his medication, she was engulfed in a haze of smoke. She watched in dismay as Big Al went into a paroxysm of coughing after exhaling a stream of smoke. Mandy warned Al that if he continued to smoke, he would make himself sick again. Al and his buddies laughed her out of the room. Mandy retreated to the nurses' station, and called me at home, bursting into tears of frustration and humiliation as she related the story. I promised to talk with Big Al first thing in the morning.

As I approached Big Al's ward, Myra, the veteran head nurse, confronted me. "Doctor, you have to do something. Things are completely out of control."

"What's he done now?"

"Last night, that room was packed with men and women, drinking and smoking and partying like they were in a South Philly strip joint. Some of the women were half naked. The place was... Anyway, this morning, your patient is coughing his lungs out, and he's really sick."

"How sick?"

"His temp is 103 degrees, and the blood tests show bad pulmonary deterioration. His oxygen content has dropped, and the carbon dioxide has risen. The anesthesiologist's already been here. He feels your patient's in jeopardy, and needs to be back in the intensive care unit, with a ventilator *and* a breathing tube. For what it's worth, I completely agree with him. You'll find it all in the chart."

The cigarette smoke had undoubtedly inflamed Big Al's raw, vulnerable lungs, and he probably had pneumonia on top of it. That would explain the fever and deteriorating lung function. I ordered a chest x-ray, a sputum specimen to check for infection, and an electrocardiogram to be certain that there had been no damage to his heart.

I was furious. How could Big Al be so stupid? I promised myself that after I examined him, I'd lay down the law. My law, for a change. I had gone along with Al, allowing him to break all the hospital rules. But breaking rules is one thing. Jeopardizing his health was where I drew the line.

Sitting up in bed, cigarette in hand, Al smiled when he saw me and took a long, leisurely drag. A violent coughing spell suddenly ensued, causing a missile of sickly green sputum to spew from his mouth onto the bed sheet. Its color was a sure sign of infection. Big Al had a bacterial pneumonia.

On the physical exam, both lungs emitted wheezes, whistles, and crackles, a dramatic deterioration from the past two days. Al was hot to the touch and flushed with fever, which according to the bedside chart had reached 104 degrees. In response to the high temperature and low blood oxygen, his heart rate had jumped from 96 to 128 beats per minute. The stress was an imminent threat to his vulnerable heart.

"Al, when we talked about the operation, you agreed not to smoke," I said in a grave medical tone. "When the nurse tried to tell you that…"

"Excuse me, Doc. You're the one who's been telling me I'm doing great. The operation's over. So what's your problem?"

"According to the head nurse, you and your friends were drinking and smoking up a storm all night. Now you have a fever, and…"

"You come in here to tell me I'm breaking some rule? Is that what you're doing?"

"No, that is not what I'm doing. Healing takes time, and the effects of the surgery and the anesthesia are *not* over. Now you're in serious danger because you just had to start smoking again. You broke your word. That's what I'm telling you."

"Hey. Watch yourself there, Doc. Don't be getting irregular with me now. KnowwhatImean?"

"Look," I said, "I'm upset. Your lungs are terribly inflamed, you have a high fever and pneumonia, and your heart may not be getting enough oxygen. None of this would have happened if you…"

"Hey, Doc. Don't give me a fuckin' speech. Just take care of the pneumonia and whatever else I got. Give me some medicine or something."

"Al, how do I get through to you? You've made yourself dangerously sick. You could die. Do you understand? Those cigarettes could do you in. The anesthesia doctor wants me to put you back in intensive care, with the breathing tube. And you know what? He's right."

"Listen to me carefully, Doc. You and him can forget about that fuckin' tube. Now don't give me any more of your doctor bullshit. Go write me a script for some fuckin' medicine."

"Doctor bullshit? Do you have any idea how hard the doctors and nurses around here have been working to take care of you? Every one of them, every shift, has given you everything they've got. We're trying like hell to get you through this, but you don't seem to give a damn. You never listen or cooperate. All you want to do is see how close you can come to killing yourself. Well, from now on, unless you're willing to work with us, I'm not going to take responsibility for you, and I won't ask anyone else around here to either."

Big Al raised his cigarette-holding hand to stop me. From the other side of the room, Freddie made a move to get up from his chair, but Al waved him back. An eternity of silence passed. When Big Al finally spoke, each word was heavy with menace.

"My whole, entire fuckin' life, nobody ever talked to me like you just did. Nobody, knowwhatImean?" Big Al paused, his steely gray eyes boring into mine. "Now, you—big high and mighty doctor—you get the fuck out of my room. Get the fuck out!"

∞

Retreating on rubbery legs to the refuge of my office, I closed the door, kicked off my loafers, and collapsed onto the sofa. My heart was pounding in my throat. Terrifying thoughts assailed me. What had I done? I had never lost my temper with a patient before. What came over me? Big Al could have me killed. What about my family? My god, this only happens in movies, not to people like me. I must be having some kind of a nightmare. I'll wake up soon and have a good laugh. Maybe if I explained it to Tony, he could fix it. He could talk to Big Al and make him understand.

Jean's buzz on the intercom interrupted my fearful frenzy. "Myra just called. She said your patient wants to see you. I guess she means Big Al."

Summoning all the courage I could muster, I made my way toward Big Al's suite like a condemned man approaching the guillotine. Opening the door, I glanced at Freddie for a sign. His face was an inscrutable mask.

"Come in, Doc," Big Al said, patting the side of the bed. "Sit over here next to me." I sat on the edge of the bed as far away from him as possible.

"Al, I don't know what got into me. I never talk that way to…"

Putting a heavy hand on my forearm, Big Al looked at Freddie. "What do you think of our friend, the doc here? Got a pair on him, or what?" Freddie nodded.

"You got some kind of balls talking to me like you did. Tony sure was right about you, knowwhatImean? You got to be a hell of a dedicated doctor to put your ass on the line that way. You really got to care about me. That took big-time cajones."

"I didn't mean to insult you. I just got upset because..."

Big Al squeezed my arm. "Hey, it's okay, Doc. You want to know what I decided? No more smoking. You got my word. Now you take care of this pneumonia thing, so I can get the fuck out of here and go home."

Reaching into the table drawer next to his bed, Al took out a carton of Camel cigarettes. "You take these. Keep them for a souvenir."

∞

After just five days off cigarettes and on antibiotics, Big Al was well enough to be discharged from the hospital. By deciding in an instant, he had stopped a lifetime of chain smoking and made another dramatic recovery.

That same afternoon, I called Tony. After some aimless chatter, I told him about my plan for Big Al's follow-up care—a good cardiologist in New York. I had done my job, and wanted out. There was a long pause on the phone.

"I understand that you don't want to be involved with Al anymore, but I promise, he will not be a problem. Al and I talked. He likes you and respects you. The most important thing is, he trusts you. Al thinks you have integrity and guts. He loved the way you stood up to him about the smoking. Al feels indebted to you, my friend."

"I'm flattered Tony, but..."

"Look, I'm telling you there's nothing to worry about. All you need to do is be yourself. Tell you what. I'll make a deal with you. Three office visits and that will be it. Okay?"

"Damn it, you always were a bulldog."

∞

Two days later, my wife called the office. "I can't believe this! Our front porch is covered with cartons of women's clothes. Dresses. Jackets. Coats—fur coats! Italian shoes. All in my size. And all kinds of toys. It's like somebody cleaned out FAO Schwartz and Bloomingdale's and dumped it all here. What in the world is going on?"

"Oh my god."

"Did this stuff come from that Big Al? Well, we are *not* going to accept it. You call and tell him to take it all back, immediately."

"I can't do that. He'll be insulted."

"Then *you* do it. Rent a U-Haul or something. The whole thing's giving me the creeps."

"I have an idea. As soon as I get home, I'll stick all the stuff in the back of the garage where no one can see it. We won't use any of the things, and…"

"You call that a solution?"

∞

When Big Al came to the office a week later, I was astonished to see how well he was doing. Again disregarding my instructions, he had proceeded far faster with his cardiac rehabilitation than I thought safe. For the past several days, Big Al had been taking half-mile walks around his beloved Brooklyn neighborhood.

Al's heart rate was a normal 88 beats per minute, the electrocardiogram was stable, and he had completely recovered from the pneumonia. But Big Al's high blood pressure had returned. His reading was considerably higher than it had been prior to the surgery, rising to 160 over 102. Since the normal reading is less than 135 over 85, Al needed antihypertensive medication. While writing two prescriptions, I told him about the disquieting development.

"Yeah, things are tough right now. Lots of shit's going down." Then, Big Al brightened. He nodded to Freddie, who went into the corridor. Two burly men, each carrying a huge carton, came into the office. "Put them over there," Al said, pointing to a corner.

"What's that, Al?"

"A little gift," he said, grinning broadly. "Tony tells me you're a scotch drinker, so we got you a couple cases of Chivas. Call it a token of my gratitude. Chivas is your favorite. Am I right?"

"You are right, Al, and I appreciate your generosity, but I really can't accept this."

"What can't you accept? A couple cases of scotch whisky? This is my gratitude, and you're saying no?" Al took a deep breath. "Damn it Doc, what's the matter with you? Take the fuckin' scotch. When I give you a nice gift, it's not respectful to refuse. When I send your wife and children some nice things, it's not respectful to hide them in the fuckin' garage. KnowwhatImean?"

So I respectfully accepted the cases of Chivas Regal scotch, with their conspicuously absent federal import seals.

I saw Big Al again a month later. He claimed to be feeling well, but his eyes were red-rimmed and puffy, and surrounded by deep, dark circles. In the interim between visits, *The New York Times* and *The Philadelphia Inquirer* had been filled with front-page stories about a rash of gangland killings. According to the news reports, a war had broken out between the New York and Philadelphia Mafia families for control of Atlantic City and its lucrative gambling enterprises. Angelo Bruno's head had been blown apart by a shotgun blast behind his ear. Chickie Narducci, Phil Testa, and a host of other Bruno lieutenants had also been murdered.

Al's blood pressure had soared to 180/108, and when I listened to his heart, the disquieting return of a gallop sound could be heard, an early sign of cardiac dysfunction. This was a potentially dangerous development, and when I began to talk to Big Al about my concern, he did something unexpected. For the first time, he ordered Freddie to leave the room.

Putting his elbows on his lap, Al leaned toward me. "You and Tony been saying that after the surgery, my ticker's stronger than it's been in years, but since I'm back, it's like my heart's not in it any more. Everything's so fuckin' hard. So much shit to deal with. I've been trying to get my organization set up to run like a legit business. A nice, clean corporate setup, with lawyers and accountants—the whole thing. The old ways aren't right, and I don't want to do business like that anymore.

KnowwhatImean? I want something better for the young guys coming up in the organization, like you want for your two children."

Big Al sighed. "But, when I called my meeting to tell them about my plan, those fuckin' Long Island goombahs look at me like I'm some kind of freak or something. KnowwhatImean? Those punks are trouble. You remember before the operation, when I told you about them?"

I nodded.

"Tough motherfuckers. Young and full of pride. Always needing to prove themselves, to show they got big fuckin' cajones. All balls, and no brains is what they got. But that shit is wrong. Used to be, I said something, and that was it. KnowwhatImean? But now they refuse to listen. Now, when I tell them, they look at me funny, like maybe Big Al, he's getting soft. I don't know, Doc. Maybe they're right.

"I'll tell you the truth. I haven't been the same since that operation, and those cocksuckers can smell it. And Doc, that definitely is not good for my health." Big Al frowned. "You got to be strong in my business. Strong like a bull. KnowwhatImean?"

"Well, Al…"

But Big Al was in no mood to listen. "Doc, just give me the fuckin' scripts."

∞

Three months later, Big Al returned for his last visit. His heart sounded surprisingly strong, and there was no trace of the gallop. And when I took his blood pressure, it had come down to 138 over 88, almost within the normal range! I had to repeat the reading to be sure it was accurate. "Looks like those blood pressure pills are really doing the job," I said.

Big Al smiled. "Know what, Doc? I never used those scripts."

"For some reason, I'm not surprised," I said, returning his smile. But I was bewildered. According to the medical textbooks, when a patient's blood pressure gets as high as Big Al's, it cannot return to normal without medication.

After I completed the examination, Al again motioned Freddie out of the room. But this time, when he interrogated my eyes, I could detect no trace of the usual menace. It seemed to have been replaced by a quiet countenance that could only be described as peaceful.

"Remember that time you came into my room in the hospital all irregular about my smoking, and I kicked you out?"

"I'll never forget it, Al," I said smiling.

"I never told you why I decided to quit."

"No, you never did."

"Well," he said, eyes still searching mine, "after you left, I thought it over, and decided I wanted to stick around. KnowwhatImean? There were things I needed to do. I had responsibilities. Lots of people depending on me.

"Something happened to me after that operation. When you doctors stuck shit into every part of my body, put me down with the gas, cracked my chest in half, spread out my ribs, and cut my heart open… Doc, you ever wake up with a fuckin' tube down your throat?" I shook my head.

"It does something to you. I've been doing a lot of thinking about things lately, Doc. I mean about the work I do. I'm not sure I want it anymore." In a wistful tone I had never thought possible, Big Al continued. "I'm going to finish up some business. Make the peace with Philly. Then I'm going home. Slow down. Take walks. I love walking, now that I don't get those pains in my chest and start coughing up my fuckin' lungs every time I go too fast. Find some peace and quiet. KnowwhatImean?

"You know something? Ever since I left my father's butcher shop, it's like I haven't had a quiet minute my whole life. Always needing to be careful. Thinking about every move. Every fuckin' detail. Peace and quiet will be good for me, don't you think, Doc? Good for my heart, and my blood pressure too. Am I right?"

"You sure are, Al."

Suddenly, his tone hardened. "Doc, you say nothing to nobody about this. Not Tony. No one."

"I won't tell a soul."

Big Al got to his feet, and gave me a bear hug. Then, holding me at arm's length, with a hand on each of my shoulders, he flashed his nicotine grin. His eyes were shining.

"Hey Doc. You take good care of yourself, and that nice little family of yours."

"You too, Big Al."

Al threw back his head, and howled. "You know, that's the first time you ever called me that? Anyway, Big Al may not be around much longer. You want to know what I've been thinking about lately?"

"What's that?"

"Maybe I'm going to get into the medicine business. Like you, knowwhatImean?"

Before I could react, my patient reached out and pinched my cheek. Then he turned, opened the door, and was gone.

∞

Soon after Big Al's last office visit, he disappeared. Some newspaper stories suggested that he had been murdered. Others speculated that he had retired, and was living in Miami or Sicily. No one seemed to know, or in Tony's case, was willing to say. When I called periodically to ask how Al was doing, Tony would say "fine," and change the subject. A strain had fallen on our friendship and after a while, we lost contact with each other.

∞

A year later, I received a newspaper clipping in the mail. It was written in Italian, but at the top of the piece was an accompanying picture showing a small group of men in white lab coats and women in nurse's uniforms standing in front of a modest one-story building. From what I could gather, the article had something to do with the opening of a medical clinic somewhere in Sicily. Standing next to the doctors and nurses, circled in blue ink, was a massive man dressed in a dark, double-breasted suit with sunglasses and a broad grin on his face. A note was enclosed:

"Hey Doc, remember when I told you I was going into the medicine business? The doctors and nurses I got here are as good as yours, almost."

"KnowwhatImean?" I said to myself with a smile.

Rosie the Riveter

"Never mind the ridicule, never mind the defeats. Open up again, old heart."
—Ralph Waldo Emerson

I like to meet new office patients in the reception area before seeing them in the more formal office and exam room settings. It helps to put them at ease, and establishes a more personal relationship. But my introduction to Rose Mirkin was unusual. As I reached down to shake her hand, the eighty-two-year-old woman looked up from her wheelchair, and commenced a complicated struggle to extricate her arms from a sea of blankets. When a mottled, blue-veined hand finally did emerge, my new patient made a tremulous attempt to reposition the plastic nasal oxygen prongs dangling uselessly from her face. Reaching out, she managed to squeeze my fingertips.

"Doctor, I appreciate your seeing an old wreck like me," she said in a weak, breathless voice. "From what my son says, you're the best physician since Myron Resnick. He was my obstetrician, so you can guess how long ago *that* was."

"Mama, the doctor has no interest in ancient history."

Mrs. Mirkin made a futile attempt to turn to her son, who was holding the back of the wheelchair, but the tangle of straps, oxygen apparatus, and nasal tubes made the task impossible.

"Howie dear, save the advice for your clients," she said, looking straight at me with striking blue eyes.

The balding, middle-aged man grimaced. "My name is Howard. I haven't been 'Howie' since I was twelve years old."

"You were Howie then, and you'll always be Howie as far as I'm concerned, even if you are a big shot lawyer nowadays."

"Pardon my mother, " he said. "She may be the most stubborn woman on the planet."

"Howie's the only reason I'm here," she said, ignoring her son. "One of the partners in his law firm is a patient of yours, and apparently you saved his life. That's what he told Howie, anyway. But I know there's nothing you can do for me. All the others say I'm too far gone."

"All I can promise is to do my best, Mrs. Mirkin." Within minutes, I had become an unwitting witness to what appeared to be a long-standing war of wills between my new patient and her son.

"Well, anything you can do to make my breathing a little easier would be welcome. I feel like I'm on a forced march up Mount Everest. And my legs look like a pair of elephant trunks."

Mrs. Mirkin's words came out in short, rapid-fire bursts, interrupted by gasps for air. But, despite being frail and severely short of breath, she seemed determined to talk. Prior to the visit, I waded through her three-inch-thick medical records. Four words had jumped out at me: "End-Stage Heart Failure."

Heart failure is a condition that occurs when weakened cardiac contractions impair the heart's ability to supply the body with enough blood to meet its needs. Unlike other abnormalities, this disorder results from other diseases. High blood pressure, heart attacks, heart muscle diseases, heart valve abnormalities, and birth defects can all cause impaired cardiac function, progressively eroding its pumping capability until the output of blood decreases.

The disorder has become a major health problem in the United States, afflicting four to five million Americans, and causing more than two million hospitalizations a year, an increase of 164 percent since 1979. Almost thirty billion dollars is spent annually on heart failure patients.

More people die of this disorder each year than succumb to breast or colon cancer. Since heart failure results from progressive cardiac weakening over many years, it is more common in the elderly, and has become the most prevalent cause of hospitalizations in people over the age of sixty-five. As our aging population continues to increase, this health care problem will undoubtedly increase exponentially.

The hallmark symptom of heart failure is shortness of breath, occurring while a person engages in physical activity. In its early stages, the weakened heart can support ordinary bodily needs, but because more oxygen is required during physical activity, it is no longer able to meet the increased demands caused by the exertion. When the heart begins to fail, edema fluid backs up into the lungs, resulting in pulmonary congestion. Once the physical activity stops, the congestion abates.

With continued cardiac weakening, shortness of breath becomes more frequent, and is brought on by less activity. Ultimately, it occurs even when the patient is sedentary. At this stage of the illness, the decreased blood supply begins to affect bodily functions. Edema fluid in the lungs persists. Afflicted patients become weak and fatigue easily. The fluid buildup no longer confines itself to the lungs, and begins to accumulate in the ankles, progressing to the legs. The liver becomes congested, increasing in size, and the kidneys malfunction.

At this stage, a patient now becomes short of breath even when lying down. To sleep, she is forced to elevate her head on two or more pillows.

While I was greeting my new patient in the reception area, evidence of severe heart failure was obvious. Even when she was not talking, her breath came in rapid, shallow gulps. While she was speaking, it was so labored that she was unable to complete a sentence without gasping for air. The blanket surrounding her hunched frame exposed ankles and feet so grotesquely swollen by liters of edema fluid that, as she had so aptly put it, they resembled "a pair of elephant trunks."

∞

"I can see the way you look at me, Doctor. It's the same as the others. All you see is a old wreck who's about to die. Tell the truth. Isn't that what you were thinking?"

"For god's sake, Mama. Can't you be a little less...?"

"A little less what? Blunt?" she said. With her eyes fixed on me, Mrs. Mirkin said, "I don't mean to be rude, but these days I skip the niceties. My breath is short and my time is running out." As if to punctuate the point, she burst into a short paroxysm of coughing.

"Mama..."

"Howie, you'll only have to put up with your cranky old mother for a little while longer, so stop telling me how to behave. Now, if you don't mind, I'd like to be alone with the doctor. Kindly wait for me outside."

Rosie sat on the exam table covered with a skimpy hospital gown, her frail frame supported by the office nurse. Parchment-thin speckled skin stretched across her forehead and protruding cheekbones, while the remainder of her face collapsed in a tired mass of shapeless folds. But also residing within was a defiant demeanor, and piercing eyes that belied her physical fragility.

"Actually, I was thinking that you remind me of my grandmother," I said after her son left the room. "Her name was Rose too. Grandma was an incredible woman—gentle and loving, but tough when she had to be."

"Is she still alive?"

"No. She died several years ago. She was ninety-eight years old."

"I'm only eighty-two, but there's no chance I'll make it to your grand-mother's age."

"Well, Grandma had some serious medical problems too. When she was ninety-one, she was rushed to the hospital with an infected gall blad-der. None of Grandma's doctors thought she had a chance, but she fooled them all. Then, when she was ninety-four, she fell and broke her hip. The doctors didn't want to operate because she was so old. They only agreed after my mother signed a consent form acknowledging the risk. Grandma came through without a hitch."

"I wish I had your grandmother's strength, but my body has aban-doned me."

"Well, let's have a look and see what we can do."

"Okay, but before you start, I'm going to ask two favors. First, I want you to promise you'll be honest with me."

I have always believed that attempts to beat around the bush or distort the truth only heighten patients' anxieties, allowing their imaginations to conjure up a host of worst case scenarios. But being honest also means not issuing absolute pronouncements that shatter patients' hopes.

The truth is that the prognosis of any illness is based on averages and statistics. No one can predict the outcome in an individual patient. Since the very nature of disease is its variability, citing cold statistics serves only to destroy hope and a patient's ability to mobilize the inner resources that can be as decisive in the fight against disease as any pill or procedure.

"Mrs. Mirkin, you have my word."

"And I'd like you to call me Rosie. I've been called Rosie ever since I worked in a parachute factory during World War II."

"Just like Rosie the Riveter."

"Do you know about Rosie the Riveter?"

"Wasn't that poster the symbol of women contributing to the war effort?"

"That's right! But you're not old enough to remember those days."

"No, but…"

"Well, it was quite a time. When the war started, my husband enlisted as a pilot, and I jumped at the chance to work in the factory. It was stupid, but I thought one of my parachutes might save…" Rosie dissolved into a coughing spasm. Shaking her head in frustration, she fought back the shortness of breath. "You should have seen me *then,* Doctor. Bright-eyed and bushy tailed, as we used to say."

"I'll bet."

"Would you believe me if I told you that I was asked to pose for one of those posters?"

"Really?"

"Yup. They made me up like a big movie star, tied a bandana around my head, and put this big rivet gun across my lap. I looked like one of those pinup girls—just like Betty Grable. Now, look at me—an old bag with a worn-out heart, and blown up like a water balloon."

"Well, you still sound like Rosie the Riveter to me."

"I don't think they ever used my likeness on those posters, but the Rosie part stuck."

"Okay…Rosie, let's take a look at you."

"Those were the days," Rosie whispered hoarsely, as I began the physical exam. "Everyone was so full of patriotic spirit. President Roosevelt told us that we were fighting to preserve our way of life. He was such a wonderful speaker. There were 'V for Victory' and 'Uncle Sam Needs You' posters everywhere." Rosie began another bout of coughing that lasted several seconds. When it finally stopped, her shoulders slumped over in exhaustion.

"Rosie, I'd love to hear more, but let's save the rest of your story for another time. I don't want you to get too tired."

My patient raised her head and looked directly at me. "There might not be another time, Doctor. I'll speak more slowly so I can breath better, but if you don't mind, I'd like to finish. I'm proud of the contribution I made to help win the war. We worked six days a week for twenty-five dollars, not counting overtime. That was a lot of money in those days. Of course, I had high blood pressure then too, but they didn't know how to treat it."

"I'd like to do the physical now. That'll give you a chance to rest, and maybe we can talk a bit more afterwards."

High blood pressure has been called "the silent killer" because it causes no symptoms, but left untreated, it can lead to heart attacks and strokes. The disease runs in families, and in afflicted patients, the arteries constrict, forcing the heart to work harder to propel blood.

In response to the increased stress, the heart enlarges and increases its muscle mass. But over time, these compensatory mechanisms become exhausted, and the heart's pumping ability becomes impaired.

Proper treatment with a restricted sodium diet, exercise, weight loss, and medication dramatically reduces the complications, but drugs were not available to treat hypertension until the late 1960s. Franklin Roosevelt himself had severe hypertension, and because no treatment was available, he too developed heart failure. In 1945, the president died of another dreaded complication of high blood pressure: a massive cerebral hemorrhage.

Rosie's chart indicated that her high blood pressure problems began in the 1940s. By the sixties, according to her medical records, her first signs of heart failure were already evident.

∞

Even when she was sitting upright, Rosie's engorged neck veins were immediate evidence that the backup of blood from her failing heart was severe. While the blood pressure was normal, Rosie's rapid pulse rate indicated that her heart was struggling to compensate for its weakened ability to adequately pump blood to her body.

When I placed my stethoscope on Rosie's chest, she jumped.

"Hey, that's cold," she said, laughing.

"Sorry," I said, trying not to show my concern about the abnormal sounds in her lungs. Coarse, bubbling sounds called rales, like those coming through a straw at the end of a drink, were present in almost a third of both lungs, indicating the presence of pulmonary fluid. Despite the oxygen being fed to Rosie through the nasal prongs, her dusky skin color was evidence of a low oxygen content in the bloodstream.

The cardiac exam was also disquieting. Rosie's heart had become massively dilated, extending past the normal point inside the left nipple line all the way to her armpit. A loud gallop sound indicated major weakness. But the most dramatic evidence of her heart failure was Rosie's swollen, waterlogged legs.

Massive swelling extended from her feet and ankles to her knees. When I briefly pressed a finger into Rosie's shin, there was a lingering indentation, a clear sign of fluid buildup. The skin over both areas was coarse and thickened.

The electrocardiogram was abnormal. In patients with hypertension, the increased muscle mass causes an increase in the heart's electrical voltage. But Rosie's electrocardiogram showed a considerable *reduction* in voltage. This indicated that much of the heart muscle responsible for generating the electrical impulses had been replaced by scar tissue, or that the ubiquitous edema fluid might have accumulated in the sac around it. Her normal cardiac rhythm was frequently interrupted by ominous premature beats.

∞

Numerous classification systems have been used to grade the severity of heart failure. The widely used New York Heart Association method grades patients from I to IV. Class I patients have no physical limitations. Those in Class II become short of breath during ordinary physical activity like walking, while Class III patients have marked limitations in physical activity. Although they are free of symptoms at rest, even walking a half a flight of stairs may force them to stop because of breathlessness.

Class IV and end-stage heart failure are synonymous. These patients are completely incapacitated. Shortness of breath may occur even at rest, worsening with the slightest physical effort. Edema fluid floods the lungs, liver, and legs. The amount of blood pumped from their battered hearts has fallen to the minimum necessary to sustain life.

The outlook for patients with heart failure is grim. One in five Class I patients die within two years, while almost half of those with end-stage disease succumb within six months.

The diagnosis on my new patient's chart was correct. Rosie had end-stage heart failure.

During the examination, Rosie seemed to doze off, but afterwards she came alive, continuing her story as if no time had elapsed.

"When the war ended, the boys came home and wanted their jobs back, so they told us to go home. Now that we weren't needed in the plants, it was somehow decided that there was plenty of work for us to do around the house."

"A woman's place is in the kitchen?" I said. Rosie was opening up, and while I was concerned that she would exhaust herself, it seemed that talking was therapeutic for her.

"Yes, and I was plenty riled up about it, but the war was over, and so was Rosie the Riveter. We all went back to our former lives and became happy little housewives again."

"In those days, I guess that was supposed to be the proper role for women, but I'm surprised you accepted it."

"Who could argue that creating a home for your children, and your husband who had just returned from the war, wasn't more important than working in a factory? So my job became doing laundry, ironing shirts, mending socks, sewing on buttons, dusting, vacuuming, scrubbing floors, food shopping, cooking, and of course, waiting on my husband and bringing up my son properly. Of course, I loved being a mother. When my Howie was little..." Rosie was interrupted by another coughing spell.

"Rosie, we need to talk about your heart problem."

"I don't like the sound of your tone, Doctor," Rosie said between gasps. "It sounds like you've got something bad to say."

"I promised I'd be honest."

"And I want you to be honest, but please try to go easy on me, okay?"

"Well, you already know that your heart failure is pretty far advanced, but..."

"But what? Doesn't that mean I'm about to die?"

Rosie the Riveter was a very sick woman, but she was also feisty and defiant. I sensed that considerable inner strength had gotten her this far, and I was not about to rob her of the hope that she could, at least for a time, beat back her disease. If she was willing to do battle, I was willing to stand with her.

"Rosie, no one can predict when you are going to die. I have patients with heart failure who have been doing well for years. There are things we can do that may improve the quality of your life."

"Frankly, these days, quality is a lot more important to me than quantity."

"I can understand that. Right now, you are on maximum doses of water pills."

"That's what the nursing home doctor keeps telling me."

"Recently, a new class of drugs has been studied in heart failure patients like you. There's no guarantee that they'll work, but they might."

"Really? Tell me about them."

Rosie's interest was a clear indication that she was not resigned to her situation. Early studies of agents called ACE inhibitors suggested that they might be effective in some patients with severe heart failure. Unlike water pills that eliminate edema fluid by enhancing water excretion from the kidneys, ACE inhibitors dilate blood vessels, making it easier for a weakened heart to propel blood into the circulation. The research also suggested that patients who responded to the drug required fewer hospitalizations, and had an improved prognosis.

But the new medication was not without risks. If Rosie's heart was incapable of responding to the more favorable environment by increasing its output of blood to the body, dilating her arteries could cause a significant fall in blood pressure. In Rosie's tenuous condition, that could be fatal. ACE inhibitors also increased the amount of potassium in the blood. If Rosie's marginally functioning kidneys were unable to adequately excrete it, life-threatening levels could result.

After I explained the situation, Rosie put her tremulous hands together and smiled broadly.

"That sounds just grand! Let's give it a go. I have nothing to lose but my life, and these days, it isn't worth much."

Rosie's response was heartening. She was ready to fight. But her son had other ideas. After the nurse and I got Rosie back into the wheelchair, they began arranging the blankets and getting her settled. As I left the exam room to order some blood tests, he cornered me in the hallway.

"Pretty hopeless, I guess," he said.

"Your mother has severe heart failure, but she's got a lot of fight in her. There are some things we can try that could improve the situation."

"Really? Everyone else who's evaluated her said that between her heart and her age, it was pointless."

"If that's how you feel, why did you bring her here?"

"To confirm that, once and for all. I thought if my mother heard it from someone with your credentials, it might finally sink in."

"What might sink in?"

"That she needs to accept her condition. I hope you're not going to give her any false hopes."

Before I could respond, Howard turned and walked off.

∞

To get an objective assessment of Rosie's cardiac function and to see how much fluid was in the sac around her heart, I ordered an echocardiogram. I also began the new medication, starting with very low doses.

The results of her echocardiogram were deeply disturbing. While the edema fluid in the cardiac sac was insignificant, Rosie's heart appeared to be quivering rather than contracting. The fact that she had managed to stay alive was miraculous, let alone managing to complete her Rosie the Riveter story.

Apparently, no one bothered to tell that to Rosie. After only a week on the new medication, she showed an unmistakable response. The most sensitive way to assess patients with severe heart failure is by weighing them. Short-term weight shifts indicate gains or losses of edema fluid. While it was difficult to detect substantial changes in the swelling of her legs by looking at them, she had lost almost twenty pounds of water weight. Most importantly, Rosie's lungs had cleared considerably, with scattered rales barely audible, and only at the lung bases. The abnormal beats on Rosie's electrocardiogram were also significantly reduced.

The change in Rosie's appearance was equally striking. Despite the oxygen prongs, she looked bright and cheery. A charming twinkle shone in her eyes.

"I feel much peppier these days, Doctor, and I don't have to sleep sitting straight up anymore. Now, I can lie on three pillows without getting short of breath."

"I'm delighted, Rosie. You certainly look much better."

"Do you really think so?" Rosie responded with a coy, flirtatious smile. "Well, if you like the way I look now, maybe you'll get a kick out of seeing what I looked like before I became an old hag." Rosie began rummaging through her purse, found what she was looking for, and handed it to me. It was a crumbling photograph album.

"These were taken when I was in my prime," Rosie said, squaring her shoulders and throwing her head back. "What do you think?"

I opened the volume, with its yellowing black and white photographs neatly arranged on black pages. On the first page, a vibrant young woman, dressed in a loose-fitting blouse and pants, with a bandana on her head, sat in a formal pose holding a rivet gun in her lap. A raised arm and rolled-up sleeve revealed a flexed bicep.

"That's my Rosie the Riveter picture. Don't I look grand?"

"Absolutely fabulous, Rosie. You look strong and confident, but feminine. Sexier than Betty Grable."

Rosie's face lit up. "No one was sexier than Betty Grable. She had those fabulous legs. But I was a real looker in those days, don't you think?"

"I sure do," I said, searching for a resemblance to the young woman in the pictures. Rosie's once dark, curly hair was now white, thin, and brittle, with furtive patches of scalp peering through. Her false teeth were prominent, and her wrinkled, receding face was now a gaunt reminder of the apple-cheeked woman of decades past. Only her eyes had trumped time. Their youthful sparkle mirrored those of the attractive young woman in the photographs.

"You certainly were a beauty," I said.

In another picture, a slender young man in uniform stood with one arm around Rosie and the other around a small boy. A third was a group picture of Rosie surrounded by coworkers. Their pride and camaraderie was palpable.

"Did you see my husband?" Rosie beamed. "So tall and handsome. I was just five-foot-one, but he was a six-footer. And how that man could dance. Before the war, when we were courting, Saturday night was dance night. Our specialty was the jitterbug. I loved the way Sammy could toss me around. He was so strong, and I felt so safe in his arms. God, I loved that man. He passed away twenty years ago, but it still feels like yesterday."

Suddenly, there was a knock on the exam room door. It was Howard.

"Can I come in? The nurse just told me Mama's exam ended a while ago."

"I suppose I'm ready," Rosie said. "You can come in."

Howard entered the room and grabbed the handles of his mother's wheelchair. "The doctor is a busy man, and I have to get back to the office. Have you been boring him with your stories about the 'good old days'?"

"She hasn't been boring me at all," I said. "I've been enjoying your family photographs."

Howard took a quick glance at the album, and frowned. "I don't know what my mother told you about those days, but our memories couldn't be more different. Mama loves to romanticize about my father, but all I remember is him sitting around the kitchen table, unshaved in a T-shirt and boxer shorts, stuffing his face with hot dogs, drinking beer, and snapping at us to bring him this or that. We waited on that man hand and foot."

Rosie began to well up. "How did you get to be such an ungrateful son? Didn't your father always provide for us? Didn't he put you through college and law school?"

Instead of responding to his mother, Howard turned and began talking to me. "He put me through hell! I got scholarships and took summer jobs to pay for school. I did it all on my own. Between his depression and her causes, I've been on my own since I was a kid."

"What are you talking about?" Rosie exclaimed. "Once I stopped working, I was always at home waiting for you after school."

"Mama's conveniently forgotten about the time she became a fundraiser for Israel."

"That was something I had to do." Rosie said, turning toward me in an unspoken plea for support. "Doctor, are you old enough to remember when the United Nations voted to create the state of Israel for the Jews, and all the Arab countries sent their armies to drive them into the sea?"

"No, but I've read about it."

"Those were *my* people over there! After the Holocaust, I wasn't going to sit at home and do the laundry while more Jews got slaughtered, so I volunteered to help raise money. It was important to me."

"You weren't a volunteer. You were a fanatic. When the Jewish National Fund asked you to be the coordinator for our neighborhood, you jumped at the chance!

"Mama rang every doorbell and got every kid in the neighborhood out on the street corners. She told us to go up to everyone who walked by, and shove the collection boxes with the blue-and-white emblems at them. I wasn't allowed to come home until my box was full, even if it got dark and I was freezing to death standing on some lonely corner."

"Blue and white were the colors of Israel's flag," Rosie said plaintively. "I was honored that they were putting their trust in me. Israel's fate depended on the money we raised for them. Without it, they wouldn't have been able to defend themselves or fight back. No one else in the world was lifting a finger to help the Jews, so we had to do it ourselves. I wanted my son to set an example for the rest of the boys."

"I know, Mama, but that's all you ever thought about. You could have thought about me once in a while. I felt like an orphan on the street. All I wanted was a little praise, a hug, some show of affection."

I felt like an eavesdropper, but was hesitant to interrupt the angry dialogue. Gaining an insight into the relationship between my patient and her son was vital to my understanding of her. But as the quarrel became more heated, they were almost oblivious to my presence. Feeling that this was becoming too taxing for my patient, I was about to step in when my pager went off.

"I'm sorry, but I'm going to have to answer this call," I said to Rosie. "Do you have any questions before I go?"

While carefully returning the album to her purse, Rosie said, "I have one question, Doctor. Do I still need these hideous plastic things in my nose? I hate them, and my breathing is so much better."

"I'm checking the oxygen content in your blood today. If it's okay, you won't need the prongs."

∞

Over the following weeks, I continued to increase the dose of the ACE inhibitor, and Rosie continued to improve. She no longer needed nasal oxygen, and was able to speak without struggling for breath. As her kidneys responded to the medication, they excreted more edema fluid and prevented the buildup of potassium in her blood. Only occasional extra beats now marred the electrocardiogram.

Two months later and forty pounds lighter, Rosie's engorged legs had shrunk sufficiently for her to abandon the wheelchair. In a demonstration of newfound independence, Rosie took a taxi to the office, and proudly entered the waiting area using a walker. But once she was in the exam room, her mood changed.

"Rosie, you've done so well. I couldn't be happier," I said after completing the evaluation.

"I'm grateful to you, Doctor," Rosie said, with a weak smile.

"Is something bothering you?"

"If you really want to know, my life is bothering me. Until now, I've been so preoccupied by my illness that I didn't notice anything else. But now that I'm feeling better, I look in the mirror every morning and think about my situation. Each day is an eternity. I have nothing to do but sit and wait for the hours to go by. I'm like the rest of the inmates at the home. I don't want to sound like a kvetch, but the truth is that we're all wasting away, waiting to die."

"Doesn't Howard visit?"

"I'm embarrassed that you had to listen to that nonsense. Howie has no time for his mother. My son's a very busy man. He got divorced recently, so he's trying to get over it by throwing himself into his law career. Just as well, if you ask me. That woman was a real witch. For some reason, Howie's always had a grudge against me, and doesn't care who knows about it. Maybe it's got to do with what he told you about the work I did for Israel. Maybe it's got to do with his father. I really have no idea."

"What about his father?"

"What Howie told you about his father was true. Something happened to Sammy during the war. He was shot down over Europe and spent a year in a Nazi prisoner-of-war camp. When Sammy came home, I hardly recognized him. He'd aged twenty years, and was a broken man. My Sammy was a complete stranger."

"Did you ever talk with him about it?"

"He told me that all of his buddies in the crew died in the plane crash, and that he was badly wounded, captured, and taken to a POW camp. But he never really talked about the effect it had on him. Sometimes, he'd wake up in the middle of the night screaming and drenched in sweat. When I reached out to hold him, he pushed me away. He completely closed off, and never wanted me to touch him. Never wanted to touch me either."

"Did you think about getting help?"

"Help? You mean like seeing a psychiatrist? In those days, no one knew about that kind of thing. Neither of us knew what to do—how to reconnect with each other. I was a passionate young woman, but when Sammy came home after the war, our love life was over. We spent the rest of our lives together like strangers. Even so, he's still in my heart. At least when he was alive, there was another human being around."

"Have you told your son that you'd like to see him more often?"

"Howie hates coming to the home, and frankly, I don't blame him. The place is a nuthouse, right out of that old Jack Nicholson film."

"One Flew Over the Cuckoo's Nest?"

"That's the one. The nurses are a bunch of Nurse Ratcheds, and the aides are a bunch of damn Nazis. They drag you out of bed and heave you into a chair, or wheel you to dinner, without even acknowledging your existence. They talk among themselves, laughing and joking about us as though we're part of the furniture. Like we're no longer members of the human race."

"Still, I'm sure it would be nice to see more of Howard. After all, he *is* your only family."

"The truth is that his visits make me feel worse. Usually when Howie comes into the room, I'm watching TV. He gives me a peck on the cheek, and before he even sits down, he's bawling me out for spending so much time in front of the tube. Tells me I should be reading a book or something. I've been a reader all my life, but I can't read in that room."

"Why not?"

"My room is like a jail cell. I share it with another inmate who complains all the time. My bed is furthest from the window, so my side gets no sun at all, and the lamp on the table between us is too dim for reading."

"Why doesn't Howard get you a better lamp? That seems like a simple enough thing to do."

"I never ask him to do anything for me, because I know he doesn't want to be bothered. There's another area where the light is better, but the Nazis won't let me use my walker. They're afraid I might fall and Howie will sue the place, so my only way out of the jail cell is to be wheeled. Of course, getting an orderly to take me anywhere requires an act of Congress. Those people refuse to do anything they don't have to do, and I'm scared to death of antagonizing them because those SOBs wouldn't hesitate to make my life even more miserable than it is already. So, you know what I tell that darling son of mine? I tell him that television is my only companion, and I feel closer to the people on the soaps than anyone in the real world. And the terrible thing about it is, it's true."

Not knowing what to say, I nodded sympathetically.

"So Howie sits there scolding, checking his watch, and looking bored and disgusted because the room reeks of urine, while I pretend to watch TV. After fifteen minutes, he gets up, gives me another silent peck, and leaves."

"Why does the room smell so bad?"

"My cellmate spends all day in bed. When she rings for help getting to the bathroom, they take so long that by the time they arrive, she's usually had an accident."

"That's terrible. Why haven't you told Howard about all that? He could speak to the administrator."

Rosie grimaced and her eyes began to well up. "Howie isn't interested in anyone but himself. I can't understand how that boy became so selfish. He was the first baby I ever held in my life. When they handed him to me, I was petrified that I would drop him. He was so tiny and fragile, with soft, downy hair on that wobbly little head and those innocent eyes. I loved everything about being a mother—the breastfeeding, changing his diapers, bathing him every night.

"When he was a boy, we'd play checkers on the living room floor almost every night. I made him adorable little costumes for Halloween, knitted him dozens of mittens and sweaters, and taught him to read and write before he went to kindergarten. When Howie was ten, I saved for about a year and bought him a bike. I even showed him how to ride it by holding him up, and running back and forth along the street a hundred times. I never got tired. In those days, I was so full of life. Having Howie was the most wonderful thing that ever happened to me. Even today, it's hard to believe that my body created a human being. Now look at it."

"Well, it's a lot better now than it was when you first came here."

"Yes, and I thank you for that. At least I think I do."

My heart went out to this lonely woman. After a lifetime of struggle and commitment to causes she cared deeply about while trying to raise a son in a loveless home, the cruelty of her isolation and the harsh reality of her life at the nursing home saddened and offended me. It seemed unjust that the woman who once was Rosie the Riveter should be forced to end her life trapped in a prison, without friends or family.

Rosie's state of mind also had medical implications. Studies have borne out what doctors have long known: Depression is a major health hazard. In a recent study to gauge depression, a thousand patients between the ages of sixty-five and eighty-five were given a standardized questionnaire called the Life Orientation Test. The most depressed group had a 55 percent higher risk of dying compared with those who were most optimistic. In the depressed patients, the death rate from heart disease was 23 percent higher.

∞

Shortly before her next scheduled visit, Rosie was rushed to the emergency room. My patient was once again in heart failure.

The scene in the emergency room was alarming. Propped up on a gurney with her head slumped to her chest and an oxygen mask over her face, Rosie attempted to get air into her waterlogged lungs by breathing in short, rapid pants. Loud bubbling noises, audible with each inspiration, were an ominous sign that they were flooded by massive edema fluid. According to the paramedics who transported her from the nursing home, Rosie had become stuporous during the ambulance ride.

A quick evaluation confirmed the severity of the sudden relapse. Rosie's circulation verged on collapse. Her blood pressure was dangerously low, and a catheter placed in her bladder revealed that she had stopped making urine.

The heartbeat had also become wildly irregular. The monitor showed a rhythm abnormality called atrial fibrillation, a disturbance that can occur when a failing heart dilates. The erratic beat added substantially to Rosie's problem, because atrial fibrillation decreases the output of the heart by as much as 25 percent.

Despite the enormous stress, Rosie's heart rate was strangely low. Whenever the heart's output begins to fall, the pulse reflexively attempts to compensate by speeding up. Under duress, some elderly patients are incapable of increasing their heart rates. But when I had originally examined her, Rosie's pulse was rapid. The low heartbeat was puzzling, but more pressing problems prevented me from dwelling on it.

I ordered intravenous Lasix to reduce the fluid buildup in Rosie's lungs, plus digitalis, a medication that both strengthens the cardiac contraction, and more importantly, can convert atrial fibrillation to a normal rhythm. Rosie also needed intravenous dopamine and dobutamine, medication to bolster her blood pressure and failing heart. But those benefits come at a huge cost. Like viciously whipping a race horse to exact its last ounce of energy before the animal collapses, dopamine and dobutamine can be used only for a short time before they cause the heart to collapse. Despite the dangers, I had no choice. Without jump-starting Rosie's heart, raising her blood pressure, and getting blood to her brain and kidneys, she would die. During the short time she had been in the emergency room, Rosie's stupor had worsened. My patient could no longer respond to simple questions.

In addition, the oxygen in Rosie's bloodstream had to be increased. The first step was to raise the percentage of oxygen being delivered through the mask to 100 percent, while doubling its flow rate.

A big question remained. If Rosie's oxygen levels did not improve significantly, the only remaining recourse was intubation. But before I took the step of putting a breathing tube down my patient's throat and attaching her to a ventilator, I needed her son's approval. Howard was waiting for me outside the ER.

As I went out to see him, a question reverberated in my mind. What could have caused Rosie's sudden deterioration? Although she had been doing well for months, the most minor occurrence could have destroyed her heart's delicate equilibrium.

The tests I ordered had already excluded infection, of either the waterlogged lungs or the kidneys. The cardiac rhythm disturbance could have provoked the relapse, or the cardiac deterioration and dilating heart could have caused the rhythm abnormality that drastically worsened the situation. Blood clots called *pulmonary emboli* could have traveled from the legs to the lungs. This too had to be excluded, particularly in a sedentary patient like Rosie.

But the most common cause of worsening heart failure was something doctors call "patient noncompliance." Heart failure patients must adhere to a low-sodium diet. One high-sodium meal, such as Chinese food or the preserved meats served in delicatessens, can be enough to precipitate a crisis in susceptible patients. Taking medication correctly is also essential. Far too often, patients are not told in sufficient detail how to take their prescription drugs. But Rosie had not been going to Chinese restaurants or delicatessens, and her medications were administered by the nurses at the home. Was this simply the result of Rosie's depression? The cause of her life-threatening collapse remained a mystery.

Howard sat in the waiting room outside the ER looking disgruntled. His reaction to his mother's situation was not unexpected.

"Sounds like the old gal's heart finally gave out."

"Howard, the situation's grave, but it's not hopeless. Your mother is a strong woman. If we can…"

"Doctor, this is hard as hell to say, but maybe it's time to let Mama go. After all, even if you manage to keep her alive, what kind of a life will she have to look forward to?"

"I don't know, but her striking improvement over the last few months tells me that she wants to live."

"What about now? Pardon me, but you don't know what my mother's life is like in that home. Mama sits in an armchair day after day, staring at a TV in a hypnotic trance. Every time I visit, she bitches at me like a crazy woman about how the people there humiliate and degrade her. You call that a life?"

"She's told me about conditions at the home."

"There's nothing wrong with that place! I pay good money to keep her there! The home's a renovated country estate in a lovely area, on acres of land. It's clean, the food's okay, the nurses are well trained, and they have a doctor who sees the residents every week. He sees Mama regularly and makes the necessary adjustments in her medication. She's well cared for there."

Alarms began going off in my head. Could the nursing home doctor have changed Rosie's medications? I had carefully evaluated the dozen or so drugs she had been taking prior to seeing me and eliminated almost all of them. But no matter how unnecessary, some doctors can't resist writing prescriptions. In our country, hospitalizations for the toxic side effects of medications have reached epidemic levels.

"I know Mama's been telling you that I never visit, but I do the best I can. My work is demanding. As a doctor, I'm sure you can understand that. And frankly, I have needs too."

"Of course. But getting back to your mother…"

"Let me make myself clear. I don't want to you making any heroic attempts to save my mother. If she doesn't respond to what you're doing, I feel we should let her go."

While agreeing to honor his wishes, I was torn. Howard feared that if his mother did not improve, I would be reluctant to remove her from the respirator. My goal was to use the breathing device only if necessary, and only to buy enough time to see if Rosie responded to treatment.

"Let's see how your mother responds to treatment. We'll discuss things again after I reevaluate the situation."

I excused myself and returned to the ER. Although she remained in critical condition, the medication had stabilized Rosie. After completing the assessment, I called the nurse responsible for her care at the nursing home and requested a list of my patient's medications.

"I'm sorry, Doctor," she said, "but we are not allowed to divulge anything about a resident's medical condition over the phone."

"Then I need the name and phone number of the nursing home doctor."

"Dr. Matthews. I have his number right here."

Dr. Matthews was no more interested in talking to me than Rosie's nurse. When I asked if he had made any changes in her medications, he said he couldn't recall. "Do you know how many patients I see over there? More than fifty a day."

"I'd appreciate it if you could look it up. This woman's life may depend on it."

"Everything is an emergency with you hospital guys." He paused. "Okay, I have it right here. Mrs. Mirkin's blood pressure seemed a little low when I saw her last week, so I cut back on the ACE inhibitor. Also, I started her on Inderal. Now, if there are no more questions…"

While ACE inhibitors do lower the blood pressure, in Rosie's case, I *wanted* to keep it low to decrease the workload on her heart. But the new drug that Matthews prescribed for her was a bombshell.

"How much Inderal did you give her?" I asked calmly.

"The standard dose. You're a cardiologist, so I assume you're familiar with the new studies about beta-blocker drugs like Inderal helping heart failure patients. Guess you didn't think a family physician like me kept up with the latest research."

The reason for Rosie's slow heart rate was now clear. Inderal slows the pulse. It also decreases the force of the heartbeat. Studies had shown that this class of drugs helped *some* carefully chosen patients with Class II or Class III heart failure, but they also demonstrated that in others, the drugs can be catastrophic, particularly in those with end-stage disease. In these patients, a further depression in cardiac function dramatically worsens heart failure by pushing vulnerable patients to the edge of a precipice. The result can be massive flooding of the lungs or dropping blood pressure leading to shock. When initiating a trial of these drugs in such tenuous circumstances, miniscule doses must be used. Dr. Matthews had misunderstood the situation. By prescribing the standard, full dose of Inderal, he made a monstrous mistake—one that now threatened Rosie's life.

"Did you know that a cardiologist was involved in this patient's case?" I asked.

"Sure. *I* certainly didn't start that ACE inhibitor. I've heard those drugs can be dangerous."

"They can be. That's why I started with small amounts. Full doses of ACE inhibitors *or* beta-blockers like Inderal can be disastrous in cases like this. Didn't you think about contacting me before starting the Inderal?"

"No. If I had to get a consultation every time I wanted to start a drug, I wouldn't have time for anything else. I'm not like you academic people. I have to work for a living. Guys like you have no idea what it's like out here in the trenches."

"Don't give me that 'in the trenches' crap!" I shot back. "You have no idea what you've done to this patient. You've put her life in jeopardy! She's had a major relapse, and is in florid heart failure. In a complicated case like this, medications have to be used with extreme care. Even small changes can…"

"Do you have any idea what that home is like? It's a shithole. The place stinks of urine and ammonia and god-knows-what. Every other patient is in diapers, so they don't crap all over themselves. Whenever I go over there, I hold my breath, do the best I can, and get the hell out as fast as I can. Now, I wish you well taking care of that woman, but if you don't mind, I have a busy schedule. Good-bye."

Rather than admit to making an error that put a patient's life in danger, this man was defiant about the shoddy care he meted out to the helpless people entrusted to him.

While waiting for Rosie's lab results to come back, I decided to redial the nursing home, and asked to speak to the administrator. This so-called doctor should have his license revoked before he killed someone. At the very least, I was going to let the person responsible for the residents know what he had done.

"I understand your concern," the administrator said in a calm voice, after I related my conversation with Matthews, "but you have to understand our situation at the home. We have a population of sick old folks here, each with their own, special needs. Most of them have multiple illnesses, requiring mountains of medications. We have to supervise our seniors twenty-four hours a day, seven days a week. I wish we could give them more individual attention, but we're on a tight budget, and for the home to stay in business, we can't afford to hire additional people. Given our limited resources, I'm proud of the care we provide our residents."

"My patient was terribly mistreated by the staff, and almost killed by your doctor."

"Frankly, Doctor, the nurses and the aides constantly complain about your patient. They tell me that she is a difficult, demanding woman."

"That has nothing to do with her medical care. What do they complain about?"

"Name it. She wants them to do things for her that she can do for herself. She's always misplacing her TV remote, ringing for a nurse's aide, and complaining that they take too long coming over to help her find it. Nonsense like that."

"I doubt that she'd ask for help if she didn't need it."

"The nurse's aides here work hard, especially since the cutbacks we had to make last year. They wash, dress, and feed most of our residents. They lift them out of bed, and clean up their mess when they don't make it to the bathroom in time. They have no time for nuisance requests. Every time the nurses at the central station look up, your patient's room light is on. When someone doesn't drop everything and run right over, she gets all upset. We do the best we can, but this isn't a four-star hotel, Doctor."

"Having a bare-bones staff is all the more reason why you need a competent, conscientious doctor."

"Dr. Matthews came to us highly recommended, and his credentials are impeccable. One of our board members referred him to us, and until this unfortunate incident, we've never had a single complaint."

"Well, you have one now."

"Of course, we do hear from family members occasionally. Some people feel guilty when they put a parent here, and making complaints seems to help them feel better. But your patient's family has never complained about her treatment at the home. Now, I appreciate your taking the time to call, and I can assure you that we'll continue to monitor Dr. Matthews' care of our residents."

I hung up still feeling furious and frustrated. For the first time, I could fully understand and empathize with Rosie's despondency. The situation at her nursing home was disgraceful.

To my astonishment, in the days that followed, Rosie began to improve. The intravenous Lasix cleared her lungs, and the digitalis converted her chaotic heart rhythm to a normal beat, enhancing her heart function sufficiently to allow us to taper off the dopamine and dobutamine. The recovery enhanced the blood flow to her kidneys, resulting in a resumption of good urinary output. Her blood oxygen content also increased, eliminating the need for a breathing tube and a ventilator. After a week, we were able to move her to the floor.

∞

Although Rosie's mental state slowly improved, the grave illness had taken a toll. When I saw her on rounds, she showed none of her usual feistiness, responding to questions in a monotone while barely acknowledging our presence. Gone was her usual spark; the glint in her eyes was now replaced by a blank stare. Initially, I thought her decline might be due to physical and emotional exhaustion, but when it appeared to be getting worse, I decided to pay a personal visit.

Rosie was sitting up in bed absently gazing at the TV when I entered the room. I pulled up a chair next to her. "Nice of you to visit, Doctor," she said, listlessly, "but you really shouldn't have bothered. I know how busy you are."

"Rosie, I wanted us to have a private chat because I'm concerned about you. After making such an incredible recovery, I thought you would be more cheerful. What's wrong?"

"My incredible recovery seems to have upset my dear son. I think he's disappointed that I'm still around. In a way, I agree with him. After all, what kind of future do I have? Between my heart and the home, just staying alive is a struggle. What's the point? Maybe it's time for me to go."

"Rosie, you've just fought off an illness that would have been fatal for most people. That tells me there must be a part of you that isn't ready to leave yet."

"If there is, it's a mystery to me. I have no idea why I'm still here. My life is like my heart: one big failure," Rosie said sadly, and began coughing so violently that she had trouble catching her breath. It seemed like a lifetime of pain was being released from her congested lungs. I moved closer to my patient and put an arm around her until the convulsive coughing stopped.

"Rosie, you've been through a terrible ordeal, but you survived. Maybe you can somehow find a way to make life better for yourself at the home."

"How? My situation there is impossible, and to be honest, I'm tired. Tired of being abused by my son, by the people at the home, and by life."

"That doesn't sound like Rosie the Riveter talking."

"I'm not Rosie the Riveter anymore, Doctor."

"Not many people could have found the courage to overcome your illness. I think that tough-minded, determined Rosie the Riveter spirit is still alive in you. She's the one who brought you through this crisis."

"Maybe you're right, Doctor, but right now, I just don't know…"

Two days later, Rosie's son called.

"What kind of nonsense have you been putting in my mother's head?"

"What? I don't know what you're talking about."

"She really unloaded on me today. When I came to visit, she wasn't watching TV, so I asked her if she wanted me to turn on the set. She said the shows are a bunch of crap, and she's seen enough. Then Mama said what she did with her time was none of my business, that she's a human being, and if I didn't start treating her like a person instead of a problem, she didn't want anything to do with me."

Bravo, I thought to myself. That's my gutsy Rosie talking! She's finally standing up for herself!

∞

On morning rounds the next day, we were greeted by a patient who barely resembled the distraught old woman I had tried to console. Her white hair was neatly combed, and a hint of lipstick, mascara, and a Cheshire cat grin gave her face a radiant look. Rosie's eyes sparkled as she chirped a buoyant "Good morning, Doctors" to our startled group.

"You look lovely, Rosie," I said.

"I decided to look nice for my doctors today, so one of the nurses helped get me dolled up."

"We're flattered."

"To be honest, I didn't do it just for you. I'm having a special visitor this afternoon," Rosie said, batting her eyes flirtatiously.

"Really? Who?"

"One of the new inmates at the home. His name is Morris. He called yesterday to find out how I was."

"How do you know him?"

"They put him at my table in the dining room. We've had some nice talks." Rosie leaned forward, and whispered, "Morris is a real looker. He's seven years younger than I am, and when I told him my age, know what he said? He said he didn't believe me, because I look so much younger! Anyway, Morris called again this morning, and wanted to know if I was up to having company. I told him that if he was up to making the trip, I'd love to see him. Do you really think I look okay? I feel like a teenager on my first date."

"Fabulous!"

Two days later, Rosie was discharged from the hospital.

On her next visit, dressed in a purple velour jogging suit, and sporting a new hair style, Rosie practically floated into the office accompanied by her walker and a tall, distinguished-looking gentleman. When I came out to greet her, Rosie proudly introduced me to her friend.

"This is Morris," she said, beaming, and then adding in a schoolgirl whisper, "Isn't he handsome?"

Smiling, Morris silently shook my hand.

Since leaving the hospital, Rosie had made remarkable progress. She was sleeping well, using only two pillows, and continuing to lose weight, an indication that her kidneys were excreting additional edema fluid. On the physical exam, Rosie's lungs were clear, her pulse was regular and beating at a normal rate, and her heart sounds were strong.

"How do you like the new getup?" she asked while I studied her electrocardiogram, confirming that her heart rhythm was normal.

"Very chic, Rosie. I think Morris likes it too. Looks like you've swept the man off his feet."

Rosie broke into a big grin. "I like Morris too. We picked this out together from one of those Sears catalogues."

"You must be spending a lot of time together."

"We sure are. Morris loves books, but he can't see too well, so I read to him. It's fun. We both love mystery novels. Right now we're in the middle of *The Little Drummer Girl* by John le Carre."

"Sounds like you're enjoying life these days. I'm really happy for you."

"It's been wonderful. Morris has a great sense of humor, and he gets a kick out of my stories about the old days. But the most important thing is, he's a sweet man. So much warmer than my husband. We can talk about things. I think he really understands me. This may sound crazy, but no one has ever understood me before. And Morris has a terrific collection of old movies. Last night we saw *Casablanca*. I just adored it." Rosie leaned over and whispered conspiratorially, "Doctor, I've never been happier in my life."

∞

But Rosie was anything but happy when she returned two weeks later. Before I could say a word of greeting, she blurted out, "You won't believe what happened this weekend. It was Saturday night, about nine o'clock, and most of the inmates were asleep. My roommate needed help getting to the bathroom, because, as I told you before, she can't get out of bed on her own. But this time, she had terrible cramps. She rang the nurses' station, but no one came. A few minutes passed, and after two more tries, she started screaming that she was in agony and needed help, and that she was losing control of her bowels. Still no one showed up.

"Finally, I got out of bed and hobbled down the hall to the nurses' station. There wasn't a soul in sight, so I began shouting and banging on the counter. After a while, the office door behind the station opened and one of the nurses stormed out, upset that I was there raising a ruckus instead of being in bed. I could see the rest of the nurses and orderlies sitting in the back room, drinking coffee, eating cookies, laughing, and kibitzing like they were having a party. I told her what was happening, and that it was an emergency.

"She said 'Go back to your room before you wake everyone in the place. Someone will be over soon.'"

"Did anyone come?"

"They came all right. After that woman had an accident, and was forced to lie in her own diarrhea for more than an hour. It was dreadful. When the nurse's aides finally did show up, they made crude jokes while they cleaned up the mess, and shoved her around like she was a sack of rotting refuse. The poor darling was sobbing with shame and humiliation."

"That's an outrage."

"You bet it is! We don't deserve to be treated like dirt just because we're old and helpless. Well, we're not going to be helpless anymore. Morris and I have decided to do something."

"What can you do?"

"We have a plan. When I told the story to the people at our dining room table, they got angry too. All the inmates have had their share of humiliating experiences. Together we figured out that thirty or forty people at the home are able-minded and upset enough about the conditions to join us."

"Join you?"

"We've been spreading the word in the dining room. Tomorrow, we're going to have a meeting, write up a list of demands, and get as many of the residents as possible to sign it. A dozen people have already said they'd come, and I think we can get at least a dozen more. We'll insist that all our calls to the nurses' stations receive a prompt response. We'll put people in the halls to make sure that when lights go on outside someone's room, that person is seen within a reasonable time. Also, we want private phones installed for everyone who wants one. No more waiting in line for the pay phone like we were at San Quentin, or having to beg the Nurse Ratcheds to use their outside lines."

"Good for you!"

"That's just the beginning. Each time one of the inmates is abused, we'll report it and insist that the offender receives a reprimand and a notation in their file. And we're going to ask for a 'three strikes and you're out' rule. Anyone who is written up three times is fired."

"Do you think they'll agree to all that?"

"Why not? It's fair. After all, we're not asking for anything that shouldn't have been done already. We want to set up a grievance committee that includes the administrator and the head nurse to review the complaints, and decide if they are valid. And Doctor, you're going to love our last item. We're demanding a new doctor to take care of us. Someone who's trained to treat old people."

Rosie's energy and enthusiasm excited me. Despite her medical condition, my patient was once again ready to do battle to change the world around her. But how could she possibly get the home to agree to her demands?

Rosie immediately noticed my concerned look. "You seem doubtful that we can do this, Doctor, but I assure you that we will. Our demands will be signed by at least twenty or thirty residents, and we're going to send it on Howie's legal stationery. If *that* doesn't get their attention, my son has promised to use his media connections to let the world know about the wretched conditions at our home. What do you think of our chances *now*, Doctor?"

"Incredible! You've come up with a great plan. Frankly, I'm surprised that Howard agreed to help you. After all, you two haven't exactly been getting along these days."

"Oh, I forgot to tell you. He came to see me last week. Stayed for over an hour."

"That must have been different."

"In more ways than one. Howie said he'd been thinking about our last conversation when I gave him a piece of my mind. Then he told me some things I never thought I'd live to hear him say. He apologized for the way he's been treating me, and said he'd like to make a fresh start."

"That's beautiful, Rosie."

"And I apologized too, for making him feel abandoned when he was growing up. And I promised not to call him Howie anymore. When I told him the story about my roommate and our list of demands, I was sure he'd laugh and dismiss it, or bawl me out for being a troublemaker, but he took it very seriously. Said he'd be happy to help us any way he could. Maybe Howie feels guilty for putting me in the cuckoo's nest in the first place, but there's no point fussing about that now."

"Maybe he could find a nicer home for you."

"I don't want to leave Morris, and besides, the residents need me. Do you know what Howie said when I told him that? He said he needed me too. He visited again over the weekend, and you'll never believe what we did. We played checkers together, just like when he was a boy."

∞

Not only did the nursing home administrator accept Rosie's demands, but as time went on, she initiated several social activities for the residents. One of her committee members volunteered to give dance lessons.

"She plays all the oldies, like *Chattanooga Choo Choo,* and *Boogie Woogie Bugle Boy*," Rosie told me. "Everyone gets dolled up like we're going dancing at the Ritz. You should see Morris on the dance floor. He's an old smoothie, a regular Fred Astaire."

"Sounds like a lot of fun."

"We have art and exercise classes too. Not that we do all that much— walk around the room, sit on folding chairs to do stretching, stuff like that. We use light weights for something they call toning, because that's supposed to be important too. But for me, it's plenty. Good heart work-out, don't you think, Doctor?"

"Absolutely."

"Maybe you should take the class too. I've read that exercise helps keep middle-aged doctors young," she said with a playful wink.

∞

Four years later, Howard called to tell me his mother passed away. After a flu-like virus swept through the nursing home, Rosie contracted pneumonia. Despite being promptly attended to by the gerontologist who had replaced Dr. Matthews, she lapsed into a coma and died soon thereafter.

As I listened to Howard, I pictured the fiery young woman in the faded photos. Rosie the Riveter worked for her country in a parachute factory during World War II, raised money for the fledgling state of Israel, and in her last years, overcame a life-threatening illness, formed a loving relationship, and led her "inmates" in a successful fight for humane treatment.

"Your mother was an extraordinary woman," I said. "I'm glad I had the chance to know her."

"Me too."

The Surgeon

*"I will preserve the purity of my life and my art,
for life is short and the art long."*

—Hippocrates

"Nurse, I need you over here, STAT."

The familiar voice thundering from the nurses' station of the surgical intensive care unit belonged to Robert Hayes Prescott, MD, chairman of the department of surgery, and director of the unit. Dr. Prescott had been at the hospital for thirty years. Now sixty-three years old, his perennial crew cut had whitened, but his handsome, chiseled face remained youthful. Dressed in his trademark custom-fitted, heavily starched blue scrub suit and spotless white lab coat, the slender, six-foot surgeon strode through his unit like a four-star general. Prescott prided himself on maintaining a schedule that would have crushed surgeons twenty years his junior.

The Chairman, as everyone called him, began rounds in the SICU at precisely 4:30 a.m. His surgical schedule commenced at six, and proceeded without interruption for the next six hours. After taking a break to see office patients for an hour or two, Prescott returned to the OR to complete his scheduled surgeries, finally ending his day by rejoining his assistants in the recovery room to evaluate the cases. He rarely left the hospital

before eight in the evening. Robert Prescott epitomized old-school dura-
bility and dedication.

∞

The Chairman was a formidable figure. When he entered a room, conversation came to a halt. When he rose to speak at staff meetings, medical colleagues cowered. Prescott had long ago mastered the art of intim-
idation, using his stature at the medical center to maximum effect.
Everyone knew that the hospital administration and its board were in
awe of the man. Over the years, he had applied his legendary surgical
skill to half of its members or their families, and the other half felt certain that the Chairman's hands were guided by a higher authority. His
every wish was delivered as a command for quick compliance. Physicians
who had known him for years addressed him by his formal name. In
turn, he referred to patients not by their names, but by the names of their
diseases.

The Chairman began rounds by declaring, "We'll start with the ulcer
in bed 2." Moving briskly from bed to bed, he issued a stream of nonstop
orders to a bevy of assistants. "Add potassium to the gall bladder's intravenous; get a chest x-ray on the lung resection; transfuse the mastectomy
with two units of blood." An underling slow to transcribe Prescott's
orders to a patient's chart would be reminded of the surgeon's time con-
straints: "Step it up. Eighteen minutes till I'm in the OR."

Prescott had the operating room suite organized in an assembly-line
style arrangement. After completing a case in one OR, he proceeded
directly to the next, where a patient waited, already anesthetized,
prepped, and draped. Postoperative care and problems that arose with his
SICU patients were relegated to his junior staff. Prescott was too busy to
be bothered by such menial chores.

It was 9:00 a.m., and the Chairman was standing at the nurse's station.
What could possibly have caused him to leave the operating room at this
hour, in violation of his sacred schedule?

"Doris, are you hard of hearing? I have a colon resection waiting
upstairs."

With an apologetic shrug, the head nurse left our rounding team at the bedside of a postoperative open-heart patient. Ducking into the treatment room, Doris emerged seconds later holding a paper medication cup, and hurried toward Prescott, now seated at the nurses' station. As she approached, the Chairman rose from his chair, grabbed the cup, and put it to his mouth.

"Why are you girls so slow?"

"Sorry, sir," Doris said.

"Next time, be more alert."

"What was *that* about?" I asked, when Doris returned to our group. Doris rolled her eyes.

Not wanting to pry, I completed rounds, and was about to leave the unit when Doris asked to speak to me alone.

"I'm not sure I should tell you this, but I'm getting worried about Dr. Prescott," she said.

"What's going on?"

"For the last couple of weeks, he's been coming down here between cases to get medication."

"What kind of medication?"

"Nitroglycerin."

"Has he been having chest pains?"

"I don't know. Dr. Prescott never says anything. But when he came down yesterday, he was short of breath and white as a sheet. About fifteen or twenty seconds after taking the nitro, he broke into a sweat and practically collapsed onto a chair."

"What happened then?"

"He sat there for about ten or fifteen minutes, got up, and went back to the OR."

∞

Nitroglycerin is standard treatment for relieving chest pains in patients with coronary artery blockages. The medication dilates the blood vessels, and decreases the work of the heart. A tablet placed under the tongue works quickly, usually relieving the pain within a few minutes.

But taking nitroglycerin for chest pain is like taking aspirin for a fever. While both drugs can decrease a patient's symptoms, they mask the disease responsible for the problem. If the Chairman were my patient, I would have insisted that the cause of his symptoms be investigated.

Of course, Dr. Prescott was no one's patient. The Chairman prided himself on not having had a physical examination in more than thirty years. In his considered opinion, they were a waste of time.

Standing at the SICU nurses' station, Doris looked at me expectantly. "Are you going to talk to Dr. Prescott?" she asked.

"I need to think about it."

I was concerned about Prescott, but if the Chairman wanted my opinion, he would have asked for it. Perhaps he was seeing another cardiologist. I decided not to pursue the matter.

I had a lot of respect for Dr. Prescott's surgical skills, but our relationship was strained. Years before, I had asked him to evaluate a fifty-year-old high school teacher who had been admitted to the hospital with abdominal pains.

"The doctor was here with his entourage," she later told me. "Without even introducing himself, he told me to pull up my nightgown. He poked around my belly for a minute or so, turned to one of his assistants, and said, 'Put this woman on tomorrow's OR schedule. We need to explore her belly. Before I could ask him a single question, he left."

"Didn't he ask you any questions?"

"Not one."

"Nothing about your symptoms?"

"No. I figured you must have told him what he needed to know."

I was too embarrassed to tell my patient that Prescott never talked to referring physicians. Instead, I opened the chart and read his consultation note. It was vintage Prescott—one sentence, written in his crimped, precise hand: "Patient needs exploratory."

Upset by the cavalier way my patient had been treated, and wanting to know what he thought about her problem, I went back to my office and called the Chairman. His response was less than gratifying.

"You've never sent me a patient before, Doctor, so maybe you don't know how I work. I'm not in the business of winning bedside manner awards. I'm an old-fashioned surgeon, but I know my job. I'm like a car mechanic. I get under the hood, figure out what's wrong, and fix it."

"Look, my patient is frightened. She could have used some reassurance."

"Of course she's frightened. Everyone who needs surgery is frightened, and there isn't a damned thing I can do about that."

"A few words of encouragement would have gone a long way. Your visit upset her."

"Words of encouragement is *your* department. That's what fancy medical school professors do—hold patients' hands and make nice."

"I don't understand why you feel that way. Even a simple gesture…"

"Professor, if you don't want to do the hand-holding stuff, send a shrink or one of the social workers they've got running around here. People with nothing better to do."

"That's *not* what I'm saying."

"I know *exactly* what you're saying. Look, yesterday, I did a mastectomy on a woman with breast cancer. When she woke up from the anesthesia, know what she did?"

"No idea."

"She kissed my hand. Couldn't stop thanking me for saving her life. And you know what? I *did* save her life."

I had heard enough self-aggrandizement and wanted to get back to my patient, but when I asked Prescott what he thought was causing her abdominal pains and why he wanted to operate, the Chairman's irascibility rose to another level.

"I have no idea what's going on inside that lady's belly. I need to get in there and take a look."

"If you have no idea, why not get an abdominal CAT scan today? Maybe it'll show that she doesn't need surgery at all."

"Professor, no one on the medical staff questions how I work, and I'll be damned if I'm going to make an exception for you. Either do it my way, or find yourself another surgeon."

"Very good advice. I think I *will* find myself another surgeon."

Despite his superb operating skills, I never again sent a patient to the Chairman.

∞

A week later, I received a page from the OR. "Dr. Prescott passed out, in the middle of a case! Please come over as soon as you can. We need your help!"

"Is he still unconscious?"

"No, it lasted less than a minute. We wanted to get him to the coronary care unit, but he insisted that he was all right and just needed to rest. One of his assistants is completing the operation."

"Where is he now?"

"In the doctors' lounge."

Prescott was in his surgical scrubs, lying on a couch, and seemed asleep when I entered the empty lounge. As I walked toward him, he opened his eyes.

"What the hell are *you* doing here?" he said.

"I know this area is reserved for surgeons," I said with a smile. "But under the circumstances, I thought it would be okay."

"What are you talking about? What circumstances?"

"One of the OR nurses told me you passed out in there a little while ago."

"I did *not* pass out! I just got a little light-headed, that's all. I was finishing my last morning case, got a little short-winded for some reason, and began breathing too fast. I probably didn't have enough to eat this morning. A little rest and I'll be fine."

∞

Fainting spells, called syncope in medical terminology, are caused by temporary reductions in blood flow to the brain. They result from a variety of conditions as innocuous as rapid breathing (hyperventilation), dehydration, or anxiety, to serious disorders, most importantly life-threatening heart rhythm abnormalities. But when a patient with cardiovascular disease faints, the likelihood of it being a major problem increases substantially. Forty percent of untreated cardiac patients with fainting spells are dead within two years.

"It would probably be a good idea for you to get evaluated."

"Evaluated? I don't have time to get evaluated. My schedule is backed up already. I have a gall bladder and a hernia to do after lunch. Then…"

I did not want to divulge what Doris told me, but there was no longer a choice.

"I saw Doris handing you a cup of medication in the SICU last week."

Prescott glared at me in silence.

"If you're uncomfortable having me look you over, one of the other cardiologists on staff would…"

"Are you hard of hearing? Look, Professor, I'm sure you mean well, but I already had one of the girls in my office get blood work. She also checked my blood pressure. Everything is fine. My cholesterol was perfect, under 200, and my blood pressure was low, only 90 over 60. Even a dumb surgeon knows that you don't get heart attacks with numbers like those."

"Has anyone in your family had a heart attack or a stroke?"

"No history of heart attacks. No strokes. I don't smoke, and I don't drink. Now, if you don't mind, I need to get back to work."

Prescott's history and lab results decreased the likelihood of his having atherosclerosis blocking the arteries supplying blood to his heart or his brain, but they did not exclude the possibility that another cardiac condition was responsible for his symptoms. A host of heart diseases can cause life-threatening heart rhythm disturbances. Birth defects, heart muscle diseases, and heart valve abnormalities can all cause fainting.

What was causing Prescott's problem? The answer could be provided only by a thorough evaluation. Clearly, that was not going to happen.

Three days later, Doris called from the SICU.

"Dr. H., please get over here as soon as possible."

"What's going on?"

"It's Dr. Prescott. He came down for a nitro a little while ago. Apparently, it didn't relieve his symptoms, because after a couple of minutes, he told me to get another one. Before I could hand him the cup, he grabbed it and stuck the pill under his tongue."

"The chest pain must have been pretty bad."

"He looked awful. A couple of seconds after that, he reached for the desk to try to support himself, but he fell sideways onto the floor and lost consciousness. There's a bad laceration behind his left ear."

"What did you do?"

"We put him into a bed, hooked him up to an intravenous, and began monitoring his vital signs. Then I called you."

"How long has he been out?"

"About ten minutes, but he's beginning to wake up. We're scared to death."

Doris was waiting for me at the SICU entrance. "He's wide awake, and trying to get out of bed."

"Let's go."

"There's something else," Doris said as we made our way across the unit. "While Dr. Prescott was unconscious, I took a quick listen to his heart. He has a murmur that sounds awfully loud."

Heart murmurs are rumbling sounds heard with a stethoscope over a patient's heart. They result from turbulence in the flow of blood as it makes its way through the various cardiac chambers. As with fainting spells, the seriousness of heart murmurs varies enormously. They can be innocuous, or can indicate a major cardiac abnormality. The location, intensity, and timing of a murmur during the heartbeat are all potentially useful clues. The physical exam was essential to determining its significance.

"Have you all gone mad? Take out that intravenous and get that monitoring crap off me!" Prescott shouted as we approached. "Doris, if I'm not out of this bed in two minutes, you, and every nurse in this unit will be history."

"Whoa there, Doctor," I said, after arriving at his bedside. "These nurses just saved your life. Lets slow down for a minute. Do you know you have a heart murmur?"

Prescott shot me a killer look. "Why can't you mind your own damned business?" Putting his free hand to the laceration, he winced. The bleeding had stopped, and it was covered with a bandage. "How the hell would I know? I haven't had a physical in more than thirty years."

"Did anyone mention it when you were younger?"

"Maybe. I don't remember. What difference does it make?"

"It could account for the problems you're having. If you'd let me listen, maybe we can get to the bottom of this."

Flashing a belligerent glare, Prescott turned away. "Make it quick."

I reached for my stethoscope, while checking the monitor screen displaying Prescott's vital signs. His heart rate was normal, as was the blood pressure at 90 over 60, but something on the screen wasn't right.

Normally, the contour of a blood pressure recording is smooth. Prescott's pressure looked as jagged as shark's teeth. This abnormality was also evident on the physical exam. The pulse in the carotid arteries of Prescott's neck was delayed, and a distinct vibration was evident, corroborating the shark's teeth appearance on the monitor. This sign, a bruital in medical terminology, is caused either by a blockage in the arteries or the echo of a murmur originating from the heart.

I put my hand over Prescott's heart. Cardiac contractions can be felt to the left of the breastbone, inside the nipple line. The Chairman's impulse felt slow and protracted, suggesting that the cardiac contractions were being met by an unusual resistance. Finally, I listened to the heart murmur.

Doris was right. The murmur sounded like a lion's roar. Its intensity peaked at the area over the aortic valve lying close to Prescott's neck. That accounted for the abnormal vibrations I had felt in those arteries.

The aortic valve is given its name because it separates the heart from the aorta, the main artery that channels blood flow to the body. When the heart contracts, the valve opens, allowing blood to enter the aorta. The heart then relaxes, and the valve closes, preventing blood from going back into the heart.

Aortic valve abnormalities are common, occurring in 30 percent of people over age sixty-five. The valve can develop leaks, but more commonly, it becomes inflamed, and over a period of decades is invaded by calcium deposits that cause it to become scarred, deformed, and rock hard. Despite all this, the valve may continue to function adequately, with the only signal of a potential future problem being turbulence in the blood streaming through, resulting in a harsh murmur—more noisy than dangerous.

But in some patients, the valve abnormality begins to partially obstruct the outflow of blood from the heart. This disease is called aortic stenosis. As the narrowing increases, the heart must work harder to propel blood through the valve. To compensate, the heart increases its muscle mass. This remarkable adaptability often keeps patients free of symptoms for many years after the narrowing has become severe. Inevitably, the heart is no longer able to compensate and symptoms occur, usually in a patient's sixties, seventies, or eighties. Eighty percent of these patients are men.

The three classic symptoms of severe aortic stenosis are chest pain, fainting spells, and shortness of breath, the latter resulting from heart failure. Once symptoms appear, a patient's prognosis changes dramatically. If a patient is left untreated, the average time to death is one to two years. Prescott had all three symptoms, and they had become more frequent and severe. That strongly suggested that his heart was no longer able to overcome the stress of pushing blood through the narrowed aortic valve.

After the physical exam, everything fit together. The murmur was typical of aortic stenosis, and the shark's tooth blood pressure contour reflected the severity of the narrowing: Turbulent blood was being squeezed through the narrowed valve. The protracted cardiac impulse indicated the extent of the effort Prescott's heart needed to propel its blood contents. His electrocardiogram indicated that the cardiac muscle mass had increased substantially. The diagnosis was clear. Prescott had a severe aortic stenosis. His prognosis was grave.

∞

"Well, Professor, time's up. What's the story?"

Prescott tried to sit up, but another episode of light-headedness forced him back onto his pillow.

"I'm sorry to have to say this, but that murmur you've had all these years is due to aortic stenosis. It's narrowed to a critical point. I'm sure you know that once patients with aortic stenosis develop symptoms…"

"Time out, Professor. How the hell do you know all that?"

"All the evidence on the physical points to the likelihood that the valve narrowing has become severe. Those chest pains, the fainting spells, and the shortness of breath indicate that it's reached the critical stage. Under the circumstances, the…"

"Points to the likelihood? You're just guessing. You really don't know squat," he fumed.

"We do need to get an echocardiogram, and a catheterization."

"While you're at it, why don't you throw in the kitchen sink? First you try to scare the crap out of me by saying flat out that I've got a life-threatening problem, and now you're telling me you need not one, but two tests to figure out what's going on. I've never heard such bull."

Sensing that Prescott was lashing out in a desperate attempt to repress the reality of the danger he was in, I tried to remain calm and reassuring.

"The echocardiogram will give us precise information about the valve and your cardiac function. It will tell us how severe the narrowing is, how much calcium has accumulated on the valve, and how much your cardiac function has deteriorated. The main reason for doing a cardiac catheterization is to get a coronary angiogram to see if there are any significant blockages. If this becomes a surgical situation, any serious coronary obstructions should be bypassed during the procedure."

"A surgical situation? You must be joking."

"If the studies confirm that your aortic valve is critically narrowed, there's no alternative."

"And if I refuse?"

"I'm sure you don't need me to tell you that without surgery, 50 percent of patients with severe aortic stenosis and the three classic symptoms die within eighteen months."

"What about the risks of *having* the surgery? Why aren't we talking about that?"

"Because you know as well as I do that the mortality rate of aortic valve replacement surgery these days is between 4 and 6 percent. There's no comparing that risk with the risk of not having the surgery."

"Well, guess what? There's no way I'm having open-heart surgery. A few years ago, my medical school roommate had a coronary bypass. They had him on the table for six hours, and when he woke up, the poor bastard couldn't move, couldn't even open his eyes. He felt like his brains had been scrambled. Said he couldn't think straight for months."

"Well, your friend might have had a bad experience, but serious problems with mental function after heart surgery are uncommon."

"Bullshit. Dying during surgery isn't what concerns me. It's what happens if those cardiac surgeons on my staff fuck up. The mortality rates you quoted so elegantly aren't the whole story, Professor. We haven't talked about the risk of my having a stroke during the procedure, or after the procedure. And what about the risk of the new valve becoming infected or malfunctioning? The number of complications following valve surgery is endless."

"You're right about the dangers of the surgery, and I understand your concerns. But the odds are that everything will go well."

"Not with those so-called heart surgeons. Those people are butchers. I never should have allowed them on my staff."

"You're a better judge of their surgical skills than I could ever be, but everyone around here knows that you've been at war with them for years, because they keep asking for more OR space and time than you're willing to give. I've been sending my patients to them for a very long time and their results have always been excellent. Of course, if you prefer, you can arrange to have the surgery done at another hospital."

Prescott leaned back and closed his eyes. "I'm not going to let anyone operate on me. I'd rather die with dignity than risk becoming a cripple or worse."

The following day, while sitting on the toilet, Prescott had a cardiac arrest. Within minutes, the hospital resuscitation team had the electric paddles on his chest, but the shock delivered to restore his chaotic heart rhythm to normal failed. The team tried again. Still no response.

When I arrived, a breathing tube was being inserted into Prescott's throat to deliver oxygen directly into his lungs. I administered intravenous medication and made another attempt. This time his heart responded. Only when he regained consciousness and became aware of what happened did Prescott agree to have the echocardiogram and catheterization.

The echocardiogram study confirmed the diagnosis. The aortic valve narrowing was severe, the valve structure completely distorted and encased in calcium. The cumulative strain on the heart was also evident. Cardiac function had become badly weakened. The only good news was that the coronary angiogram showed no significant coronary artery blockages. This decreased the risk of surgery.

After discussing the results of his tests, I again pointed out that the odds for his survival were far better with an operation.

"Yes, but you're forgetting what we talked about," he said.

"What's that?"

"The odds of my becoming an invalid are higher if I have the surgery."

"That's not necessarily true. The next cardiac arrest could result in a stroke, or irreversible brain damage."

"There's no need to be so blunt, damn it. I get the picture," he snapped.

A breakthrough at last. Citing the cold, hard facts seemed to have penetrated Prescott's wall of resistance, so I shifted gears.

"This is tough stuff, and I know I'm coming on strong, but we've run out of time. The bottom line is that if you agree to have surgery, your chances of living a normal life are excellent."

"My life is my work."

"I know that, and there's every reason to think that you'll be able to continue working after the surgery."

"You're a persistent SOB, Professor. Okay, let's do it. I'll be damned if I'm going to lie here waiting for another cardiac arrest. The sooner I get this over with and get back on the job, the better. Just make sure those surgeons you're so crazy about don't screw up."

∽

Two types of artificial aortic valves can be used to replace a diseased one. Each has advantages and disadvantages that need to be carefully discussed in detail with every patient. But when I broached the subject, Prescott said, "I don't want to talk about it. Do what you think is best."

Prescott's refusal to participate in such a vital decision was totally out of character. His obsession with control seemed to be melting under the fear of the unknown. Having made the decision to have the operation, Prescott seemed resigned to whatever fate had in store. Reluctantly, I selected the valve, while doing my best to make him comfortable with my reasons for the choice, before going ahead with the operation.

∾

The procedure went well, but following its completion, a serious problem arose. Two hours after being moved to the recovery room, Prescott remained unconscious. All of his vital signs were normal, as were his heart sounds, and there was no evidence that his new valve was malfunctioning. Air moved normally through both lungs, and blood studies revealed normal oxygen levels.

Some patients are slow to recover from the effects of anesthesia, and since no other problems were evident, there seemed no reason for alarm. The attending anesthesiologist concurred.

But after another hour went by and Prescott still remained unconscious, my anxiety began to build. Nothing had changed on the physical exam, but I decided to get an echocardiogram to more accurately evaluate Prescott's heart and new valve. The test confirmed that everything was in order. The heart ejected blood normally, and the new valve opened and closed perfectly.

My concern now shifted: Prescott might have had one of the dread complications of aortic valve surgery that he feared. Perhaps the procedure *had* caused a stroke or brain damage. I asked the chairman of neurology to evaluate the situation. His exam revealed nothing to suggest brain malfunction. The heart surgeon, anesthesiologist, neurologist, and I conferred and all agreed that the most likely cause for Prescott's persistent unconsciousness was the persistent effect of the anesthetic.

Two more hours passed with no change. Massive brain injury now resurfaced as the most likely diagnosis. The neurologist ordered a CAT scan of the brain. To our collective relief, it was normal. Still stymied, I decided to go over my patient one more time. As I bent down to listen to his heart, I felt Prescott's hand on my forearm. He had finally awakened.

Relieved, I was now certain that everything would now proceed routinely. That did not happen. Prescott's level of consciousness fluctuated wildly. At times, he seemed awake and alert, though unable to speak because we had to keep a breathing tube in his throat. Then, he would unaccountably lapse into what seemed like a coma, becoming unresponsive to his surroundings. The anesthesiologist was certain that the drugs he had administered during the surgery had been excreted hours ago. Neither the neurologist nor any of the doctors involved in Prescott's care could figure out what was taking place.

The following morning, the situation remained unchanged. Once again, we repeated the tests, including another brain scan. Again, they were normal. Then a thought came to me.

During the two days prior to his surgery, Prescott exhibited strange behavior. He lashed out bitterly at the indignities of being a patient. The proud Chairman was infuriated at being forced to submit to nurses, lab technicians, and orderlies—people he had always considered underlings. Finding himself subjected to their insistence on taking around-the-clock vital signs, and blood and urine samples, while enduring a stream of dutiful well-wishers from the hospital board and the medical and administrative staffs, only made him retreat further. His snarling and snapping became so fierce that a joke began circulating around the hospital that the people taking care of the Chairman needed to get rabies shots in case they were bitten.

Prescott avoided his humiliating situation by turning off the world. I tried to restrict the unnecessary intrusions, but his embarrassment intensified when it was time to be prepped for the operation. The Chairman found himself naked to the world, having his body shaved, laxatives administered, and a catheter inserted into his penis. During this massive assault on his self-esteem, Prescott became so withdrawn that the staff was barely able to communicate with him. I wondered whether the current situation could be a continuation of that behavior. Certainly, depression is not uncommon after surgery. Later that afternoon, Prescott seemed a bit more awake, so I set out to give him a status report, letting him know that the worst was over.

"Your heart is strong, and the valve is functioning perfectly," I said. "Everything points to a rapid recovery. Once you complete rehab, you'll be back doing surgery again."

Prescott signaled for a pencil and paper, scribbled a note, and handed it back to me.

"Guess the butchers did okay."

Recovery now progressed rapidly. We quickly weaned Prescott from the respirator, and removed his urinary catheter. Soon he was able to take enough food and fluids by mouth to allow us to do away with his intravenous and move him out of the SICU.

As the Chairman's postoperative recovery accelerated in the privacy of his own room, his preoperative persona reasserted itself. During rounds, he buried his face firmly in the pages of a loose-leaf notebook, scribbling furiously in defiant silence, his eyes radiating anger alternating with aloof indifference as we poked, and prodded, and probed his heart.

One afternoon, as I began to write a routine note on Prescott's chart, one of his nurses came over.

"Have you heard the latest? A couple of hours ago, Dr Prescott called his office and ordered one of the secretaries to bring the SICU floor plan to his room immediately. Then, he told us to stay away because he's busy and doesn't want anything to interrupt his concentration. Now, every time we go in, he throws a tantrum and kicks us out."

"The SICU floor plan? What in the world is he doing with that?"

"I have no idea. He keeps looking at the drawings, shaking his head, and scribbling furiously in that thick notebook of his. The man must have half the pages of that thing filled up by now."

The following day, despite the Chairman's edict not to be disturbed, my curiosity finally got the better of me, and I decided to make a spontaneous visit. Ignoring the hand-lettered sign in bold print that read KEEP OUT, I knocked on the door of his private room. After several raps, I heard the thunderous growl.

"Go away!"

"It's the Professor," I said, opening the door a crack. It was a bright fall day, but Prescott had the blinds drawn. The room was steeped in darkness, save for a ray of light that escaped from a small reading lamp adjacent to his bed. Propped up on pillows, Prescott kept his nose buried in a large loose-leaf notebook as I entered.

"Can't you read, for Chrissake? I've already been poked and punctured fourteen times today."

"This is just a little social visit, to see how you're feeling since your transfer from the unit."

"I'm too busy for courtesy calls. Come back next month."

"I understand you've been looking over the SICU floor plans. Are you thinking about making some changes?"

"The SICU has to be completely overhauled. The place is a nightmare. The lights are too bright. I had to stay on my back day and night, and couldn't sleep a wink. There's absolutely no privacy. You have to lie there helpless and exposed to the world, while every damn doctor, nurse, and orderly goes about their business like you don't even exist. We need lights with dimmers, and individual cubicles for each of the patients."

"Sounds like a great idea."

"It's more than a great idea, Professor; these changes are essential. I'm working on a totally new design. We're going to install video cameras to maintain maximum patient observation. As soon as I finish my floor plan, we'll get a formal architectural rendering, price it out, and get to work. I've already dictated memos to the administrator and the board chairman."

"That's going to be pretty expensive."

"The hospital board will do what I ask them to do."

I did not have to remind the Chairman that he was the one who had designed every detail of the current SICU. He had *wanted* it to be a large, open space, brightly illuminated by fluorescent lights. The nurses and several staff surgeons had voiced concern about the lack of patient privacy, but Prescott had insisted the only thing that mattered was that each patient be clearly visible from the nurses' station. The hospital's intensive and coronary care units had video cameras installed in each patient's room for this purpose. Prescott argued that in his unit, it was unnecessary and a waste of money. As always, the Chairman had his way.

"I guess your perspective has changed," I said.

"Maybe it has."

"If you don't mind my asking, what else have you been putting in that notebook of yours?"

"I'm working on a training manual for the SICU personnel."

"Really? I've always felt that your people are very well trained."

"Maybe they know what to do medically, but they have a lot to learn about taking care of people. Those nurses don't have a clue about what their patients are going through. They just jab and prod your bodily parts as casually as if they were inspecting a slab of beef in a supermarket. Never a word of encouragement or sympathy for what a patient might be feeling."

"Maybe they were trying to be casual to avoid embarrassment. After all, you were still their boss."

"It wasn't just the way they treated me. The other patients were treated the same way. The girls aren't callous; they're oblivious. Not a single, solitary one understands what a patient experiences after surgery—the vulnerability, the embarrassment, the uncertainty."

Had Prescott forgotten that he had handpicked the SICU personnel? Perhaps the Chairman was incapable of accepting responsibility for creating the atmosphere that he had found so repugnant in his own unit.

When I visited Prescott on rounds the next morning, the room was still blanketed in darkness. Before beginning the physical, I opened the curtains slightly. The sunlight poured into the room, illuminating a table of get-well cards and baskets of flowers.

"Close the damned curtains," Prescott said, shielding his eyes from the sun.

Overnight, the Chairman seemed to have resurrected his forbidding façade. Moving toward the window, I searched for a way to break through to him.

"You know, I've always thought that surgeons are remarkable people."

"Really? Now why in the world would you think that, Professor?"

"Only a special kind of person has the boldness, self-confidence, and skill to cut into a human body. One minor misstep can be fatal. I've never understood how you deal with the fear of making that mistake."

Prescott removed his hands from his eyes. "It's a discipline, Professor. You learn to lock up your emotions, shut out everything, and focus on the job. I know I'm a Neanderthal, but I cannot understand the kids going into medicine today. I was brought up to believe that being a doctor was a total, twenty-four-hour-a-day, seven-day-a-week commitment. It came with the territory. We had this quaint idea that doctors were supposed to be dedicated.

"These days, doctors don't want to get their hands dirty, and they'll do anything to avoid being called in the middle of the night. The only thing these so-called doctors are interested in is lifestyle-friendly nine-to-five jobs that pay big bucks, like radiology and dermatology."

"Or cardiology?" I said.

"You said it. I didn't," Prescott said, betraying the hint of a smile. Talking about medicine seemed to have awakened something in the surly surgeon, and he was finally opening up. Seeing how the passion for his calling brought him to life, I marveled at the shift.

"Not too many cardiologists would agree with you there," I said, returning his smile. "Most of our patients have their heart attacks in the wee hours. But no one I know could keep up with your schedule for long. I sure couldn't."

"It's about being completely committed, Professor. I've always said that if you want a life, don't become a surgeon. But after *this*," he said, pointing to the bandages over his chest, "I'll never be able to maintain that same pace."

"Maybe that's not such a bad thing. It'll give you a chance to develop other interests."

"My only interest is surgery. It's the only thing I know, and the only thing I've ever wanted to do, since I was a kid."

"Why did you want to become a surgeon?"

"Because I wanted to be like my father. He was a family physician in Harrisburg, Pennsylvania, and his work was his life. Everyone revered the man, and so did I. Going with him on house calls made a huge impression on me. My father's patients looked at him like he was a god. When he was examining them and his fingers pressed into their neck or aching abdomen, or even when his tongue depressor made them gag, I could see the trust and the gratitude in their eyes."

It was as if a dam had been broken. All the pressure that Prescott had locked within himself now poured out in a torrent. The once aloof, supercilious Chairman was animated and engaged. His story fascinated me.

"Pretty powerful stuff for a young boy."

"It was. Those memories are etched in my mind. After the house calls, my father would return to his office on the ground floor of our home. By the time he arrived, the waiting room was packed with patients—mothers with squealing children, disabled war vets, bawling colicky babies. The patients kept pouring in, and my father never stopped. He'd see up to ten patients an hour until about six, have a quick dinner with the family, and start all over again. When evening hours finally ended, he'd go out to make more house calls. The man wouldn't get home until ten or eleven at night."

"That's unbelievable. Just hearing about it is exhausting. I see where you get your commitment and stamina."

"It didn't end there. Around midnight, the phone started ringing. I could hear my father from my bedroom. Inevitably, the hall light would go on, and then there'd be tramping down the stairs, the sound of the car starting up, and off he'd go."

"How'd he manage to keep that pace? It must have taken a terrible toll."

"The man was incredibly strong. He never complained, never seemed to get tired, never got sick, just kept on going day after day, year after year, until finally he worked himself to death."

"How did he die?"

"One evening during dinner, my father winced and grabbed his back. When I asked him about it, he said that nothing was wrong. But the pains continued and soon they became so severe that he couldn't stand up straight. One night, I heard him start down the stairs to make one of his house calls. Suddenly there was a scream and a loud noise. I raced over and saw my father lying unconscious at the foot of the staircase.

"My mother called an ambulance, and it rushed him to the hospital, but he never came around. The doctor taking care of him told us that the fall caused a cerebral hemorrhage, and that he also had a huge mass in his abdomen. I'll never forget watching my father lying in a coma under an oxygen tent. I stood at his bedside and made a silent vow to carry on his work. About an hour later, he was gone. The autopsy report said that in addition to the cerebral hemorrhage, father's cancer had spread through-out his abdomen, invading his liver and lungs."

As the Chairman's icy countenance continued to disappear, and the glowering glacier that had encased him began melting away, his face filled with emotion. Emerging before me was a vulnerable human being.

"Then why did you decide to become a surgeon instead of a family doctor?"

"One day, when I was about ten or eleven, my father decided to remove a wart from my hand. When he drew up the local anesthetic into a syringe with a huge needle and began injecting it into my hand, I closed my eyes. My father told me to open them. 'How will you become a doctor if you can't watch a minor operation?' he said. I was his only child, and my father just assumed I'd go into medicine. Until then, I'd never thought about it. I wanted my father to be proud of me, but the whole thing intim-idated me."

"What happened then?"

"When my father was ready to inject my hand, I held my breath while he stuck the needle into the area. The injection made the thing swell up like a gum ball. Then, he put down the syringe, picked up a stainless-steel scalpel, and started slicing through the skin and peeling back the flesh surrounding the wart. Bright red liquid oozed from the cut. The sight of my own blood and raw flesh shocked me. I felt myself become nauseous and light-headed. Finally, I passed out.

"Of course, my father was terribly disappointed in me. After that, he kept questioning whether I had the stomach to be a doctor. But I was determined not to let him down. I'd have walked barefoot over a bed of hot coals to please that man."

"Didn't that mean becoming a family physician?"

"My father was frustrated by his inability to provide better treatment for his patients. He drilled it into my head that those magic elixirs he dispensed from his black doctor bag were close to worthless. Nothing he could do for his patients changed the outcome of their diseases; it just made them feel better. According to my father, surgeons were the only doctors who did anything worthwhile. His pronouncements about the value of surgery made an indelible impression on me. I knew I had to become a surgeon. It was an obsession."

Prescott was discharged several days later.

∞

After one week at home, the Chairman returned to work, throwing himself into his SICU renovation project. He pored over the architect's renderings, scrutinizing every detail, making endless modifications, and insisting on twenty-four-hour turnarounds.

The cubicles had to be of precise size, and of material that screened out all extraneous noises. The position and angle of each video camera was studied to make certain it would provide clear patient observation while not being intrusive. The lighting had to be outfitted with dimmers, and had to provide indirect illumination.

Also during this time, distressing dreams began to disturb his sleep. He told me about one of them after an office visit.

"I was up all night trying to repair a liver that had been lacerated in a car accident. I tried everything I knew to patch the damn thing up, but blood kept seeping out of it. As you know, it's almost impossible to get stitches to hold in a liver after it's been badly mutilated. After what seemed like an eternity, knowing the patient wasn't going to make it, I closed the abdomen and left the OR."

"How did you feel?"

"There was no time to feel anything. My next case was waiting, and I had to go back to work. As soon as I opened the abdomen, a massive tumor confronted me. It was everywhere, like an octopus, invading and strangling all the vital structures. Everyone in the OR realized that the cancer was inoperable, but I was determined to get as much of it out as possible. So, I'm cutting away, and becoming more and more fatigued, while everyone is staring at me like I'm a madman. Hours pass. By now I've been in the operating room for who knows how long, and I'm so exhausted that one of the nurses begins to feed me through a straw."

"Were you able to finish the operation?"

"Finally, but I couldn't completely remove the cancer."

"What happened to the patient?"

"That's the worst part of the dream. After the surgery, he became dependent on machines to stay alive. The family, everyone begged me to pull the plug, to stop everything, turn off the machines, and let him go, but I couldn't. I insisted on keeping the man on a respirator, putting his family through hell. But he wasn't the only one. I kept working, kept cutting people open, kept finding that there was nothing I could do for them, and kept putting them on respirators. After a while, there were rooms full of patients on respirators. Finally, they hooked me up to an intravenous so I could keep going.

"These dreams are driving me crazy. I have no idea what they're about. Hell, I can't remember ever having a dream in my life before this."

"They're only dreams," I said. "In real life, you help lots of patients."

"You're damned right I do. Know what I think? The dreams are telling me that I need to get back into the operating room ASAP."

The following afternoon, I was in the SICU seeing a patient and noticed several nurses in a huddle, whispering and laughing.

"What's that about?" I asked Doris.

"Dr. Prescott made SICU rounds this morning for the first time since his surgery."

"I can't imagine that there'd be anything funny about that!"

"You should have been there. Dr. Prescott begins by asking who was in the first bed, and one of his assistants says, 'Oh, that's a routine gall bladder.' Well, Prescott loses it! He starts going off about calling patients by their diseases rather than their names. He gets beet red and his veins start bulging out of his neck. 'What's my name?' he says. 'Am I the aortic valve? Am I?' Finally, Dr. Prescott stops and storms out of the unit. The whole thing was incredible. If that man doesn't get back into the OR soon, he's going to have a stroke."

Everyone fully expected the Chairman to make a triumphant return to the OR. But several weeks went by, and while continuing to make daily SICU rounds with his staff and seeing office patients, Prescott still had not performed any surgery.

Finally the day came. Word went out from the department office that Prescott had scheduled a procedure. Everyone in the hospital, from the medical staff to the janitors, knew that the Chairman was back. Two days later, Prescott called, wanting to see me as soon as possible.

"I can't do it anymore," he said.

"Can't do what?"

"Operate. Ever since my surgery, I've been dreading the OR, but I knew that sooner or later I had to get myself up there. So, as everyone seems to know, I scheduled a patient for a hernia repair. Real kindergarten stuff. I began to scrub, and my heart started pounding. The patient was already anesthetized, prepped, and draped, and when I entered the OR, my team was ready and waiting as always. Believe it or not, they actually seemed happy to see me. One of the nurses gowned and gloved me, but as I walked toward the table, the pounding became worse, and I began to have trouble breathing. It felt as though I was being suffocated by my face mask, but I was determined to keep going. I asked for a scalpel, made my incision, and began cutting through the soft tissues to expose the field around the hernia, while my assistant cauterized the bleeding blood vessels. Suddenly, the smell of burning flesh hit me, and I began to feel dizzy."

"Was it anything like the faintness before your surgery?"

"It was nothing like that. This time, I didn't feel light-headed. Everything began to spin out of control. The patient, the table, and I were all revolving around like a top. I handed the scalpel to my assistant, and told him to continue while I observed. The spinning finally began to slow down, but there was no way I could complete the operation. After a few minutes, I walked out of the OR. The minute I left, the spinning stopped."

"Why did you wait two days to see me?"

"I knew that what happened had nothing to do with my heart surgery. It was nerves. I figured it was my first time back, and once I completed a case, everything would be fine."

"You scheduled another case?"

"Early this morning. A patient that needed a simple lymph node biopsy. But this time, I couldn't even make it to the OR. The spinning began while I was changing into my scrubs. I got so dizzy that I almost fell into my locker. It's over. My career is finished."

Sorrow-filled eyes and the furrows appearing on Prescott's forehead betrayed his attempt to mask the pain.

The following day, he resigned his position as Chairman of the department of surgery.

∞

A month later, Prescott came to the office for a routine postoperative visit. He had no cardiac symptoms, and showed no evidence of anguish about leaving the hospital. The physical exam confirmed that his new heart valve was functioning normally. After I completed the evaluation, we met in the consultation room.

"Well, you're certainly doing well from a medical point of view. How are you spending your time these days?"

"I've been trying to figure out what to do with myself now that I can't do surgery anymore. I was getting nowhere. Then, a couple of weeks ago, I had another one of those dreams."

"What was it about?"

"I was making rounds in the intensive care unit with my father. A child in a coma had just been admitted to the unit. Father walked by, looked at the boy, and continued on to the next bed. When I asked why he didn't do anything for the patient, my father said that he was too far gone, and that nothing could be done. 'Come along,' he said. 'We need to spend our time with patients we can help.'"

"Did you obey your father?"

"I lingered at the foot of the boy's bed, just staring at him. When I saw his face, I realized that the child was *me*. My father called for me to catch up. There were patients waiting who needed to be seen. But something stopped me. For the first time in my life, I disobeyed my father, and in that moment, I knew I had to heal that sick little boy."

"What did the dream mean to you?"

"I no longer need to blindly follow my father's dictates. And before I can take proper care of patients, I need to take care of myself. Surgery wasn't what excited me about becoming a doctor. It was those house calls with my father. He wasn't the epitome of warmth and compassion, but his commitment to them came through. His presence gave them hope. When I woke up, I realized that as a boy, I saw the effect a caring doctor could have on a patient. Now I want to recapture the calling that inspired me to go into medicine."

"What do you have in mind?"

"I've decided to start a family practice."

"That's a great idea! You can send me all your cardiac referrals!" I said laughing.

"We'll see about that," Prescott said with a wry smile. "It'll depend on how nicely you communicate with my patients."

"Touché," I said, remembering our infamous confrontation over the schoolteacher I had asked Prescott to see years ago.

"When I didn't wake up right after the surgery, I know you and the others thought the operation might have scrambled my brains. Maybe it did, in a way. I want my patients to relate to me as a person, not as a medical authority, so I'm going to have them call me by my first name. I want them to feel cared about as well as cared for, not isolated and intimidated."

"Doctor Bob?"

"Has a nice ring to it, don't you think?"

∽

"Dr. Bob" blossomed in his new calling. As his practice and reputation for compassionate care grew, patients flocked to him, and medical students began to request that he serve as their proctor. When his enthusiasm and charisma resulted in more applicants than he could handle, the medical school dean prevailed on Bob to teach a course on patient-doctor relationships.

Bob invited patients to share their personal experiences. After staff psychiatrists and psychologists were enlisted to teach the art of communication, each student was videotaped during mock history-taking sessions with patients. Later, Bob and his self-conscious students laughed together while they critiqued the tapes in class.

"How about simply smiling when you introduce yourself?" Bob would say. "A warm handshake. Eye contact. It'll put your patient at ease, and who knows? Maybe you'll relax too."

The course grew to include research documenting the value of prayer and the uses of meditative and alternative practices in healing. It became a model emulated by medical schools throughout the country.

Over time, Bob and I became friends. We met regularly in the hospital cafeteria for coffee or lunch, sharing patient stories and talking about our hopes and dreams, and the future of health care.

One day after lunch as Bob headed back to his office, he turned and said, "Remember that sick little boy in my dream?"

"Sure, what about him?"

"He's getting better every day."

Mom

*"For extreme diseases, extreme remedies. For other disorders,
the most exact therapy is best... .First, do no harm."*

—Hippocrates

It was a late Friday afternoon, and I had just finished returning the last of my phone messages, when my secretary buzzed the intercom.

"Sheila is on the line," she said. I took a deep breath before picking up the phone. Sheila was my mother's housekeeper.

"Oh, Doctor, this is so awful. I am so sorry! When your mother and I talked on the phone last night, she sounded fine." Sheila began to sob.

"Sheila, try to stay calm. Just tell me what happened."

"I came in to clean the condo like always, but it was so hot in there, I could hardly breathe. I checked the thermostat and it read 120 degrees."

"What about my mother?"

"Your mother was lying in bed. At first, I thought she might be asleep, but when I tried to wake her up, she didn't move. I called 911 right away. The paramedics just took her to the hospital."

I could feel my heart pounding, but a lifetime of confrontations with life-and-death emergencies had taught me to become calm and focused during a crisis—to suppress all emotions. My mother lived in Rancho Bernardo, a town north of San Diego. It would take me about three hours to drive down from Los Angeles.

"Where did they take her?"

"I don't know. It's that hospital near here. Oh god, I can't remember what it's called."

"Did the paramedics leave a note with a name or a phone number?"

"Yes, they did. It's right here—Palmeros Community Hospital, on San Bernardo Road."

I scribbled down the telephone number, and after thanking Sheila, dialed the hospital, got connected to the ER, and asked for my mother's doctor.

After a few minutes, a male voice came on the line. "I'm Dr. Long. Your mother's in critical condition and frankly, I don't think she's going to make it. She's in a deep coma—totally unresponsive. Her blood pressure's barely obtainable, and we've had to use high doses of medication just to get it to barely acceptable levels. And, in the last twenty minutes, her breathing's become erratic. We need to intubate her—put a tube into her windpipe so a mechanical ventilator can breathe for her. If we don't do it immediately, she'll die."

"Please go ahead. I'm a cardiologist, so I understand what intubation is, and why she needs it."

"When she came in, her temperature was 108 degrees. We have no idea why, but we're lowering it as quickly as we can. What can you tell me about your mother's medical history? Does she have a thyroid problem? I was thinking this could be what we call 'thyroid storm.' That can cause extremely high fevers. I already called a thyroidologist to..."

"It's heat stroke. I guess the paramedics didn't tell you, but my mother's housekeeper said the thermostat in her condo was 120 degrees."

How could such crucial information not have been communicated to the ER doctor? This lapse could have resulted in a fatal misdiagnosis. But I did not want Dr. Long to know I was upset. He might decide that I was going to be a troublemaker.

"My mother's been very healthy," I said. "She's eighty-six years old, but..."

"Eighty-six? Look, I'm not sure we should proceed with the breathing tube. The chances that an eighty-six-year-old can survive this are less than one in a thousand. Plus, at that age, she's almost certainly suffered irreversible brain damage by now."

"I know my mother's old, but she's had no health problems. She lives on her own, and thoroughly enjoys her life. Let's give her a chance. If she doesn't come around in a day or two…"

"Look, I think you're making a huge mistake, but I can't pull the plug without your approval."

"A day or two is all I'm asking for."

"What medications is she taking?"

"None."

"No medications? I've never heard of an eighty-six-year-old on no meds. Well, we'll do what we can, but I have to be honest. She's making no urine, her vital signs are terrible, and at eighty-six…"

∞

As I was driving down on the 405 freeway toward San Diego, my mind was racing faster than the car. Heat stroke. Just weeks before, an early summer heat wave had taken the lives of more than seven hundred seniors in Chicago. The elderly are particularly vulnerable. When their temperatures rise, they are less able to eliminate heat from their bodies than younger people. Once their temperatures exceed 106 degrees, the brain cells quickly become affected. The result is coma, along with what the medical textbooks call "multiple organ system failure."

Mom was a classic case: coma, shock, kidney and respiratory failure, and who knew what else. Lab studies could reveal liver damage, or a breakdown of her red blood cells, coagulation system, or muscles. The list was endless. Dr. Long sounded like he knew what he was doing, and I knew he was probably right about Mom's chances. The situation seemed hopeless.

But Long did not know some important details that were in my mother's favor. Mom had good genes, a resilient body, and a strong will. Her mother, my grandmother, lived a healthy, vigorous life until she died in her sleep at age ninety-eight. And Mom had already fought off two life-threatening illnesses earlier in her eighties.

At age eighty-two, Mom overcame septicemia, an invasion of a particularly virulent strain of bacteria in her bloodstream resulting from a kidney infection—an illness that is often fatal in patients half her age. Two years later, she went into shock and almost died of a massive hemorrhage in her GI tract, caused by the side effects of the over-the-counter drug Advil.

When her doctor remarked, "Your recovery is miraculous, especially for someone your age," Mom fixed him with her all-too-familiar glare.

"That's because *you* thought I was just another feeble old lady. But believe me, Doctor, I'm the toughest damned cookie you'll ever meet."

Certainly *I* needed no reminder of that. In my childhood years, Mom was a five-foot-one-inch fireball whose blue eyes blazed with the ferocity of Attila the Hun as she set about the task of molding her two children. My gentle father had christened her "the drill sergeant," because she continuously drilled the message into our heads that life was combat, obstacles were challenges to be overcome, and nothing was more loathsome than being a loser. For her children, winning meant becoming a success in life. Life was about survival of the fittest, and Mom was obsessed with instilling that Darwinian fire into an indolent son who was content to spend his time playing ball and hanging out.

My resentment toward my mother had tempered through the years, and as time passed, I came to appreciate her. Mom loved words and ideas, learning, and classical music. Since the death of my father fourteen years before, she spent her days in Rancho Bernardo reading two or three books a week and doing countless crossword puzzles, while blasting her favorite symphonies and operas on the stereo. And she continued to be preoccupied with another of her lifelong passions—politics. Her fierce nature showed no sign of mellowing with age. Mercifully, she reserved most of her venom for the politicians on CNN and C-SPAN.

In recent years, my mother and I had often talked about life and death. "I'm perfectly prepared to go," she said, "but I do love life. The workings of the world continue to fascinate me, and I adore my family. Of course, I've never been a religious person. Your grandpa and grandma were strict Orthodox Jews, but it felt too oppressive to me. In those days,

I was a pretty strong-minded rebel. These days too, I guess. It's always been my nature. I'm always raving and ranting at God to right the wrongs of the world. It never does any good, but *someone* has to say *something* about those politicians.

"I can't get over how complacent people have become. No one cares about anyone but themselves anymore. It's infuriating. If you ever saw the way I curse at the TV screen, you'd think I was a left-wing lunatic."

"No, just my mom."

∞

As the glass doors to the Palmeros Community Hospital swung open, Dr. Long's comment about the odds of Mom's having irreversible brain damage were still weighing on me. What if she neither recovered nor died? Would I know when to let go? In all likelihood, there would be little need to worry about that.

I managed to retain my composure while the emergency room receptionist casually consulted a computer printout. "Your mother's been transferred to the intensive care unit. It's through the double doors to the left."

"She's still alive!" I thought, entering the hospital corridor.

At the ICU entrance, I was confronted by two stainless steel doors. Feeling as if I were standing before a sanctum sanctorum, I was momentarily immobilized, and had to brace myself before pushing the metallic square on the wall. Slowly, the doors separated, exposing a brightly lit unit consisting of two rows of curtain-enshrouded beds on either side of a nurses' station replete with the requisite maze of monitor screens, computers, chart racks, and phone banks. For me, units like this were as natural a habitat as my living room, yet I found myself struggling to keep from feeling overwhelmed. What must it be like for those distraught families unfamiliar with this alien world?

∞

"My name is Dr. Helfant," I said to a uniformed nurse who had been suspiciously eyeing me. "My mother is a patient here." Returning to her magazine, the woman pointed absently to her left.

Slowly parting the curtain surrounding Mom's bed, I surveyed the scene. Amid a labyrinth of tubes from numerous IV bottles, bleeping blood pressure and EKG monitors, and the intermittent sighs of an artificial ventilator, my mother lay unconscious, her face sunken and arms extended at her sides, palms up, as if in prayer. A man in a lab coat with his back to me, assisted by a nurse with a tray of surgical tools, had cut open my mother's wrist and was inserting a tube into an artery. They looked up at me warily.

"I'm the patient's son," I said.

"The doctor is doing a procedure on your mother," the nurse said. "Please wait in the visitors' room. He'll talk to you as soon as he's finished."

"Thank you," I said, and retreated. Moments later, I joined the ranks of the anguished, anxiously awaiting the unknown in the windowless visitors' room.

∞

"I don't have time to go into detail right now, but I'm going to give it to you straight. Her chances are lousy," Dr. Long told me two hours later. "She's still in a deep coma. Her fever's down, but her blood pressure is at dangerously low levels despite megadoses of powerful drugs. We're pouring fluids into her intravenously to correct the severe dehydration. I've got lines in an artery, several veins, and a flotation catheter in her heart, but she's not breathing on her own, and her kidneys are completely shut down."

"I appreciate your being so direct, and I want to thank you for taking such good care of my mother. I'm a cardiologist, so I know what you're doing and why. Okay if I see her now?"

Dr. Long nodded gravely. There was no need for him to remind me that he thought I should pull the plug, as doctors call it—shut off the respirator, stop the IV, and let Mom go.

My initial instinct was simply to be a son, to sit by my mother's bedside, and hold her hand while the doctors took care of her. Despite the cacophony of bleeps and heaves from the machines that were keeping my mother alive, she looked remarkably peaceful. I had that to be thankful for. But my instincts proved too strong, and I soon found myself taking a medical inventory. While it confirmed Dr. Long's analysis, my conclusions left a bit more room for hope.

The lab results showed that there had been no liver or muscle breakdown, and Mom's red blood cells and coagulation system were intact. If any of those elements were damaged, her situation would have been hopeless. This also meant that the cause of the shock, with its attendant low blood pressure and kidney failure, was due solely to massive dehydration. I looked at the intravenous drips. As Long said, they were wide open, pouring desperately needed fluid back into her circulation.

If the amount of circulating blood was increased quickly enough, Mom's blood pressure should improve, enhancing the delivery of life-giving oxygen and nutrients to the kidneys and most importantly, to her oxygen-starved brain.

This undoubtedly was an overly optimistic scenario, but I knew my mother. Her toughness and resiliency had been tested before and she had prevailed. But this was her ultimate test. The next several hours would be critical.

I tell my students that in medicine, direction is everything. A blood pressure of 90 is a danger signal if it has previously been 120, but if it has come up from 60, 90 indicates improvement. Countless times I had stood watching patients hover at that perilous point. Some turned the corner and went on to live, while others deteriorated and died. Mom was now at that crossroad.

At midnight, a nurse named Roz entered the cubicle, and told me she would be taking care of Mom for the next eight hours. "It's late and you look exhausted," she said, and gently suggested that I check into a nearby Travelodge. "I promise I'll call if there are any changes in your mom's condition, and I promise to take good care of her too." Those were the kindest words I had heard all day.

I found the motel, phoned my sister in Connecticut and my two adult children in Denver to tell them what had happened, and crumpled into a fitful sleep.

∞

When Roz saw me entering the Palmeros ICU at six o'clock the following morning, a smile spread across her face.

"Your mother's improved. We've corrected her dehydration and her blood pressure's much better. She's requiring less dobutamine and dopamine to keep it at normal levels. And her kidneys have opened up a little. Not much urine yet, but something at least."

"That's great. What about the coma?"

Roz grimaced. "No change that I could see. She hasn't moved at all. Never responds when I talk to her or poke her arm. I'm sorry."

"That's okay. You did a wonderful job and I'm grateful. Has Dr. Long come in yet?"

"Oh, I forgot to tell you, from now on Dr. Doleman will be your mother's doctor. He and Dr. Long rotate every few weeks between this ICU and a larger unit in El Centro a few miles from here. Dr. Doleman likes to start early—he should be here any minute."

This was disquieting news. I had not seen Dr. Long again after his dire half-minute summary of Mom's condition, but I liked his treatment plan. How competent would this new doctor be?

Sitting on the edge of Mom's bed, I took her limp hand in mine, and whispered in her ear. "Mom, can you hear me? Can you squeeze my hand? Blink your eyes?" No response.

Did the brain swelling that caused Mom's coma result in irreversible damage, or had her nervous system managed to remain intact, preserving itself in a state of hibernation for as long as possible until its blood supply could be restored? This is what the heart does when it has been put in jeopardy by a coronary artery occlusion. Now that Mom's blood pressure had increased, time became the vital factor.

As I straightened up, the respirator caught my eye. Yesterday, it was triggering Mom's every breath. Now *she* was triggering the machine. Mom's ability to breathe on her own had returned! Could this be the first sign that her coma might be lifting? Direction is everything. If things continued to improve, if no setbacks occurred...was it possible...

Suddenly, I felt a tap on my shoulder. I turned to face a short, intense-looking man in a starched white lab coat who appeared to be in his late thirties.

"I'm Dr. Doleman. I'm taking over Mrs. Helfant's care," he said in a brisk, unmistakably New York accent. "I'll have to ask you to leave while I evaluate her."

Anxious to establish rapport, I held out my hand and smiled. "Your accent sounds familiar. I'm a cardiologist in Los Angeles, but I'm originally from New York."

Dr. Doleman grabbed my fingers in a perfunctory handshake. "Look, I need to go over your mother. Then we can talk."

Pretty stiff guy, I thought, sitting alone in the deserted visitors' room, which was littered with empty soda cans, candy wrappers, half-eaten sandwiches, and outdated newspapers. Why do so many of us mask our insecurities with a gruff authoritarian mien that intimidates patients and their families? It begins in medical school when we first confront an actual patient—a live human being, not a cadaver or a disease under the microscope.

Once students go on the wards, they are introduced to a macho environment where far too often bravado substitutes for compassion. Wanting to fit in with the senior physicians, they unwittingly develop a false persona and a condescendingly can-do swagger. Each student understands that he must appear knowledgeable, even when he is clueless and ridden with anxiety. I have always taught my students that it is okay *not* to know. That none of us really knows all that much. That we would all be better doctors if we were more honest.

Right now, I wanted Dr. Doleman to feel more comfortable with me. I knew he was uptight about my being a doctor. How could I gain his confidence and trust? About an hour later, he came into the visitors' area and gave me his assessment, rapidly ticking off each item.

"Your mother's a sick lady. She can't breathe. She can't generate a blood pressure, and her urine output is zilch. I'll try to keep her alive over the weekend. If she manages to make it to Monday, we'll do an EEG to see whether or not she's brain dead. If she is…"

"I understand, and I can see that you're doing everything possible for her," I said, thinking that this guy needed a crash course in Tact 101. "I know she's in good hands. By the way, I detect a familiar accent. *Are* you from New York?"

"Yeah."

"Did you train there?" I tried.

"Yeah. Beth Israel."

"Really? Did you know Fred Posner, the chief of cardiology there?"

"Yeah."

"Fred trained with me back when I was at Penn. He's a good man."

"Very good. You trained him? What do you do in LA?"

"I'm chairman of cardiology at Cedars-Sinai." Immediately, I realized my mistake. In an attempt to find common ground with Dr. Doleman, I succeeded only in intimidating him. Quickly, I tried to repair the damage.

"Look, I don't want to get in the way of your taking care of my mother. I know she's very sick, and that it could go either way."

Dr. Doleman looked at his watch. "You'll have to excuse me. I have other patients to see."

Despite Doleman's dire assessment, my medical intuition told me that while there had been no breakthrough, things were improving, and there was reason at least for hope. Returning to the ICU, I began my routine check of the monitors around Mom's bed. Suddenly, I sensed something drawing my attention to the bed. I looked down, and met my mother's eyes. They were wide open, staring in the silence broken only by the blips and bleeps of the machines.

"Mom, it's me," I said, too loudly in my excitement. "Do you know who I am?"

She nodded, and began to move a tremulous hand toward the breathing tube. Gently, I put my hand over hers. "There's a tube in your throat. It's there to help you breathe. You've been in a coma, but you're getting better. Much better."

Amy, Mom's nurse on day shift, entered the cubicle. "Well, hello there. You woke up. How wonderful."

Mom began to edge her hand toward the tube in her throat.

"No. No," Amy said. "You can't touch that. You're on a ventilator. You absolutely cannot touch that. Understand?" Mom nodded. Her hand slid back to her side.

"How much dobutamine and dopamine is she on?" I asked.

"She's off the dobutamine, and getting only tiny amounts of dopamine."

"Fantastic. What are her breathing parameters? Maybe she'll be ready to be weaned off the ventilator in a couple of hours."

Amy stiffened. "It would be best if you discussed that with Dr. Doleman. He's a pulmonary specialist, and he has strong feelings about ventilators. He'll be back in about an hour."

Waiting for Dr. Doleman, I was so elated, I actually felt hungry. Having been responsible for taking countless patients off ventilators after open-heart surgery, I knew when and how to remove them.

After a patient is judged capable of breathing on her own, removing a ventilator is done in stages—a process called weaning. First, the ventilator is removed from the patient's breathing tube while she is given oxygen-enriched air through the tube. The patient's breathing rate, and the amount of air she is able to inhale with each breath, are monitored. Those two parameters are the key guidelines, although other measurements, especially the oxygen and carbon dioxide levels in the blood, can also be helpful. If the breathing rate and the volume of air taken in with each breath remain in the normal range over several hours, the tube can be removed. A repeat check of Mom's breathing pattern showed that she more than met the criteria for successful weaning.

∞

Two hours passed, and when there was no word from Dr. Doleman, I presumed that he was caring for another patient in the hospital. By now, Mom had begun to give me that familiar glare, as though I'd brought home a B on my elementary school report card. Pointing to her throat, she tried to speak, but couldn't because of the tube.

"I know you're uncomfortable, Mom."

Mom shook her head emphatically.

"Try to be patient. Dr. Doleman should be here shortly. As soon as he arrives, I'll ask him about removing the tube."

Mom moved her head up and down in concurrence, and closed her eyes.

When Amy returned to the nurses' station at two o'clock, I asked her to page Doleman. It was becoming late in the day and I was sure that if he were available, he would want to be around while Mom was being weaned. Since she regained consciousness, her breathing pattern had remained normal.

"Do you know if he's tied up with another case?"

"He isn't," Amy said with an embarrassed look. "I'm sorry, but we have orders not to page the doctor unless there's a medical emergency. He gets really upset."

"I don't want to interfere with the way you do things around here, but my mother is really uncomfortable. All the parameters indicate that we can at least try to wean her, and I'm sure Dr. Doleman will agree. If you want, tell him I'm bugging you, so he'll blame me. I'll leave the unit. Say whatever you want."

An hour later, Amy came out to the visitors' room. "Dr. Doleman just returned my page. He told me to tell you he'll be down when he can, and…" Amy paused and lowered her head, "to stop bothering the ICU nurses." Grinding my teeth to keep from saying something I would regret, I returned to Mom's cubicle.

As I opened the curtains, a frightening scene confronted me. Oblivious to my presence, Mom stared straight ahead frantically blinking her terror-filled eyes, while twisting and contorting her body and head. Something was terribly wrong.

I quickly checked the monitor. Mom's heart rate was elevated, but her heart rhythm and blood pressures were both normal. The respirator was functioning appropriately, and its connection to the breathing tube had not kinked or been disconnected. Mom's blood oxygen content was also normal. Nothing seemed amiss.

As I looked down at the bed sheets to see if any of the lines, tubes, and electrodes had gotten misplaced, the bedside railings began to rattle.

Removing the sheets covering Mom's arms, I found the cause for what was happening. Both of her wrists had been strapped to the railings. In an attempt to communicate the source of her distress, Mom was jerking at the rails.

Putting my hands on hers, I said, "Mom, try to calm down. I'm going to take care of this right now." After she nodded, I stormed over to Amy. "What's going on?"

"What do you mean?"

"Why have you put restraints on my mother?"

"Oh, that," she said, sounding relieved. "We were afraid she'd pull out the breathing tube. No big deal. We use restraints all the time."

"Have you ever stopped and thought about what it must be like for a patient?" I asked. "You're wide awake. You're able to breathe, but there's a tube in your throat and a machine controlling your every breath. And when you try to get help, someone ties your hands down. Now, you can't speak or breathe for yourself, and you're immobilized. You can't move or communicate at all."

"I don't like the idea of restraints either, but with out-of-it old people, sometimes we have no choice."

"First of all, she is *not* out of it. And secondly, what does age have to do with anything? Please remove the straps. I'll make sure she doesn't touch the tube."

"Tell me something, Doctor," Amy asked evenly, as she complied with my request, "have you ever ordered restraints on your patients?"

Amy had hit a nerve. Of course I had—innumerable times—oblivious until now of the effects it could have on a patient.

At 3:30 p.m., Dr. Doleman strolled into the unit, and I immediately shifted gears. Despite my upset at what seemed to be his casual handling of my mother's case and the needless discomfort it was causing her, I did not want to offend him. I was a family member, and *he* was the doctor. He was in control, and my mother's fate was in his hands. There were no other options. Dr. Doleman was the only qualified ICU physician at Palmeros Community Hospital. Swallowing my feelings, I put on a smile. How many of my patients and their families had smiled at me in the same way, despite boiling with frustrations and resentments similar to what I now felt?

"I gather your mother's waking up," he said without breaking stride. "I'm going to evaluate her. Please wait outside."

"If you don't mind, I'd like to talk to you about…"

"After I've looked things over, I'll let you know what I'm going to do."

Chastened and angry, I once again withdrew to the visitors' room. A pattern had developed. Whenever things got uncomfortable for either the doctors or the nurses, the solution was to make me disappear. It was another practice I had often resorted to. Striding up and down the hallway outside the unit, I had now become upset at myself, and at doctors everywhere, for our insensitive treatment of patients and our unwillingness to speak openly and compassionately to a patient's loved ones, simply because it was more expedient to banish them to the Siberia of the visitors' room.

After I was allowed to return, Doleman acknowledged the obvious. "Your mother's made good progress today. Frankly, I'm amazed. For a woman her age to come around like this is….I'm stopping the dopamine. Her kidneys are wide open."

"What about the respirator?"

"Your mother's not a candidate for weaning today. It's too late in the afternoon. She's become agitated, so I'm going to reinstitute restraint orders. We'll keep her well sedated and assess things in the morning." He turned and began walking toward the door.

A composite picture of every elderly patient I had ever cared for on an artificial respirator flashed through my mind. In twenty-five years of practicing hospital-based medicine, how many of them had I unnecessarily sedated?

Sedation might be necessary when a patient is uncontrollably agitated. But how often was this done because of a hypothetical concern that a patient *might* become agitated, or simply because taking the time to calm a troubled patient might take too much of the busy doctor's time? A sedated, docile patient might be easier to deal with, but how dangerous was this practice, particularly in the elderly?

Brain dysfunction, swelling of the larynx, and potentially life-threatening bacterial lung infections are the most obvious risks of sedation. What effect does sedation have on an already traumatized patient's spirit? How many of the elderly end up on permanent life support because of an arbitrary medical decision that numbed or depressed their ability to mobilize those inner resources so essential for recovery? Could anyone really know? I sure didn't.

Of course, in Mom's case, I could well have been wrong. Doleman was a pulmonary specialist, and he had a more objective view of Mom's situation than I did. But why the need for sedation and restraints? It certainly seemed reasonable for us to talk about these matters.

"Dr. Doleman, I'd appreciate it if we could discuss your decision," I called out.

Snapping around to face me, his dark eyes narrowed. "Look, you've been pestering me and my staff all day. I know you're a doctor, and I know she's your mother, but she's *my* patient. This is a judgment call, and I've made the judgment." When I began to speak, he stopped me.

"Do you know how you'll react if your mother crashes when we pull the tube and we can't get it back in fast enough to save her life? I'll tell you what most people would do—sue the hell out of my ass, that's what. Now back off and let me do my job."

How could I find a way to communicate with this man without making it seem to him like a clash of egos? "Please understand. I'm not questioning that you're my mother's doctor, or that I may be too emotionally involved to make the best call here. I'd just like to talk about it for a minute."

Looking at his watch, Doleman let out an audible sigh. "Fine. Go ahead. What's your problem?"

"My mother has made an incredible recovery. You said so yourself. She's wide awake and the respirator is making her very uncomfortable. We'd both feel the same way if we were in that bed. Most important, her weaning parameters have been solid all day long. They indicate that it's safe to..."

"I am a trained pulmonologist! Dealing with respirators is what I do. What do you know about it? Cardiologists have no experience with respirators. Just let me do what I've been trained to do."

"I'm not questioning your expertise. I've had a fair amount of experience with respirators, but that's not the point."

"That's exactly right," Doleman said. "The point is that I'm the doctor here, and you're going to have to respect my decisions."

The time had come for me to confront reality. Mom was not going to be weaned from the respirator today. I decided to plea bargain about the sedation and the restraints.

"All right," I said, "but I'd appreciate your not sedating and restraining my mother. I'm sure I can make her understand that she has to keep her hands away from the breathing tube."

Crossing his arms, Dr. Doleman stared impatiently at the ceiling as I plowed ahead. "I'm sure you're as concerned as I am about the risks of sedating elderly patients. We both know that even in small doses, the effects of these drugs on their consciousness levels and their breathing patterns can be unpredictable. My mother is even more vulnerable because she's just come out of a coma."

"Do you think you're telling me anything I don't already know? Damn it, I don't have time for this."

In desperation, I hardened. "I'm going along with you about the respirator," I said, looking into his eyes. "Now I'm asking you not to sedate my mother."

"Fine. If that's what it takes to get you off my back, the hell with it." Wordlessly, Doleman turned and left.

Roz was back on duty when I returned to the unit. "Dr. Doleman just canceled the sedation order. He said you insisted. And don't worry about the restraints. Your mom and I understand each other. I'll keep her calm. That's the main problem—when patients wake up and realize they have no control over their breathing, they can panic."

"You are an angel," I said, wanting to hug her. Once again, Roz was reminding me how invaluable a competent, compassionate caretaker is to a patient's recovery.

∞

At six the next morning, Roz had just turned Mom's care over to Amy when I came into the unit. "Your mother had a great night," Roz said, beaming. "I just love her. She relaxed and didn't fight the respirator the entire night. That really took courage."

Mom smiled through the tube as I bent over to kiss her cheek. "Sounds like Roz has become a fan of yours," I said. "Everything's on track." Mom brought her tremulous hands together in a sign of victory.

As Roz prepared to leave, Mom took her hand and blinked in silent gratitude. She knew that this caring woman had saved her from a night of hell, and a possible medical setback.

When Doleman finished his ICU rounds, Amy informed me that he had ordered another set of blood studies before making a decision about removing the tube. I was unconcerned. When the tests came back thirty minutes later, they were perfect. Absolutely normal. There were no more impediments to removing the tube.

At 1:00 p.m., Doleman strode into the unit, glanced at Mom's blood study reports, told Amy to start the weaning protocol, glared at me, and left.

Mom was weaned from the tube without a hitch.

"Thank God they finally got that awful thing out of my throat," Mom said hoarsely when I returned to her cubicle. "What took them so long? If not for that darling girl…"

"I'm sorry you had to go through that," I said.

"What happened to me?"

"Your condo overheated. You've been in a coma due to heat stroke. If Sheila hadn't come in when she did…"

"God was keeping an eye on me."

"I guess so."

"Remember what I told that arrogant doctor the last time I almost died?"

"Sure do."

"Well," she said smiling, "looks like your old drill sergeant mother is still a pretty damned tough cookie."

As the elated but exhausted patient closed her eyes for a nap, and I began to leave the unit for a late lunch, I noticed Amy emptying a syringe into one of Mom's intravenous bottles. "What's that?" I asked casually.

"Oh, your mother's Doppler study showed deep vein thrombosis in her legs. The doctor ordered a blood thinner."

Deep vein thromboses are blood clots in the leg veins. They are not uncommon in elderly patients who have been bedridden for any length of time, because prolonged inactivity causes blood in the leg veins to stagnate. The main danger of these clots is that one or more pieces can break off, travel through the bloodstream, and lodge in the lungs—a potentially fatal complication called a pulmonary embolism. The best way to prevent them is by using anticoagulants—medications that decrease the ability of the blood to clot. These so-called blood thinners prevent clots from getting larger, and make them less fragile and less likely to break off.

But blood thinners are two-edged swords. Because they inhibit the blood's ability to coagulate, these drugs can sometimes cause bleeding that can vary from superficial bruises to a serious internal hemorrhage. To minimize the danger of excessive blood thinning, their effects on coagulation are monitored with blood tests.

"What happens now?" Mom asked when I returned.

"My guess is that Dr. Doleman will want to keep you in the ICU for another day or two. After that, you'll go to the main part of the hospital. They move patients through pretty quickly these days."

"Priorities sure have changed since my day. Anyway, the sooner I can get out of here, the better," she said.

But four days after her recovery, Mom remained in a weakened state. She needed assistance getting out of bed and into a chair, and still required medical supervision to regulate the dose of her blood thinner. Palmeros had a convalescent facility adjacent to the main hospital called The Villa. It seemed ideal for Mom's rehabilitation. Doleman agreed.

"I want to keep a close eye on those blood clots," he said. "Most doctors around here are pretty blasé about them, but as a pulmonary physician, I know what the risks are."

With Mom out of the woods medically, and my sister, Lucy, having just flown in from New York to provide emotional support, I drove back to Los Angeles to catch up on my patients at Cedars-Sinai.

When I returned three days later, Mom was happily situated in The Villa, already getting out of bed without assistance and navigating the corridors with a walker. She loved their food, and according to my sister, was in great spirits, having become mother hen to the entire nursing staff on the floor. I asked Lucy for a medical update.

"What has Doleman told you about Mom's blood clots?"

"Actually, Dr. Doleman hasn't seen Mom. I guess he's pretty busy at the hospital. My pal Abe, the head nurse here, confided that doctors get reimbursed for only one visit a month when their patients are at The Villa."

"That could be one explanation," I deadpanned. "But Doleman made a point about wanting to keep a close eye on those clots."

I went to Mom's bed and leaned over for a kiss. "Things are looking great, Mom. You've come through like a champion."

"Can't complain about a thing," she said with a hug. "I just love the people here. They're warm and friendly, and they treat me like a queen."

"That's because you *are* a queen."

"How about we do a couple of crossword puzzles? I need to get my brain going. I've been feeling light-headed and exhausted all day."

Straightening up, I noticed something on the underside of Mom's left upper arm. It was a black and blue discoloration, the size of a grapefruit. Alarms went off. The bruise could be a sign of more widespread bleeding—a complication of the blood thinner.

"I'd like to take a quick look at your tummy," I said calmly. One glance confirmed my fear. My mother's abdomen was covered with huge black and blue blotches. Gently, I reached around to feel Mom's flanks, a common site of internal bleeding. A giant mass of blood had accumulated there, seeping through the tissues to the skin. The bleeding was widespread. No wonder Mom was fatigued and light-headed. I rushed out to see Abe at the nurses' station.

"Are you aware that my mother has large collections of blood all over her abdomen and in her flanks?"

Abe was startled. "No. The nursing staff doesn't examine patients in this facility."

"Who does?"

"The doctors."

"Has anyone checked her blood work?"

Abe shrugged.

"I'd like to see my mother's chart. She's probably getting too much blood thinner."

The goal of the medication is to thin the blood so it coagulates one and a half to two times less readily than normal. The dose Mom was receiving was so excessive that it had thinned her blood to more than three times normal. No wonder she was bleeding.

What was Doleman thinking? I needed to talk to him. After he picked up Abe's page, and I told him what happened, there was a long pause on the line.

"Your mother's too old for anticoagulants," Doleman said flatly. "She's too sensitive to the medication. We're going to have to do a surgical procedure on her. She needs a Greenfield filter implant."

I could not believe what I was hearing. "My mother's age is irrelevant, and she's *not* sensitive to the blood thinner. All she needs is a lower dose. I've looked at her chart. The doses have varied all over the place, and her blood tests are way out of whack—more than three times normal. You've probably been too busy with your patients in the ICU to…"

"Who gave you permission to look at my patient's chart?" Doleman shouted into the phone. "Look, the pharmacy's responsible for prescribing the dose of your mother's anticoagulant. That's the way it's done at The Villa. Anyway, the dose is beside the point."

"Beside the point? That *is* the point! My mother doesn't need a Greenfield! All she needs is for you to follow the blood tests yourself, and get her on a stable dose of thinner that'll keep it in an appropriate range."

"I've had it with your constant interference. You're not letting me do my job, and I'm going to put a note to that effect on your mother's chart."

It was certainly true that without some form of treatment, Mom was in danger of developing a life-threatening pulmonary embolism. This put me in a terrible quandary. If she were to become seriously sick again, Doleman and his group were the only intensivists caring for critically ill patients at Palmeros Community Hospital. Dare I risk antagonizing him by finding another doctor? If so, how would I go about it? I did not know the medical community at Palmeros. Fearing the unknown, I decided on another approach.

"I'm perfectly willing to take responsibility for the decision to keep my mother on a lower dose of the anticoagulant, and have it in writing on her chart. If she bleeds again, I'll concur with the Greenfield operation. Write whatever you want, and I'll sign it."

Doleman was silent. Maybe he was rethinking his decision. Maybe he was thinking of a potential lawsuit. Maybe he wasn't thinking at all—just reflexively acting to cover up his mistake. I had seen *that* often enough.

"Here's what I'm going to do," he said. "I'm putting her on a lower dose of thinner. But I'm also going to write a note about all of this in the chart. If anything happens, if your mother has an embolism and dies, you'll be held responsible."

"Fine."

∞

Oblivious to my struggles with Dr. Doleman, Mom remained cheerfully preoccupied with her crosswords. She was on a hot streak: three completed *New York Times* puzzles in a row. Shortly after I joined her, a lab technician came into the room and asked Mom to roll up her sleeve so she could take a blood sample. I asked what test she was getting. "A type and cross-match. Dr. Doleman ordered two blood transfusions."

"Why do I need a blood transfusion?" Mom asked.

"You've had some internal bleeding because of the blood thinner medication. Try not to worry. I'm sure…"

Mom looked at me incredulously. "After everything I've been through, do you really think a little bleeding is going to worry me? *Nothing* is going to stop me from going home to my life."

Another check of the medical chart showed that Mom's stools had tested strongly for blood. She was bleeding into her gastrointestinal tract, and as a result was dangerously anemic. Her red cell blood count had dropped to less than half normal. Apparently, Dr. Doleman knew nothing about this until now.

Mom was scheduled to get the transfusions at eight the following morning. At nine, I called the nurses' station from my motel room to be certain she was upstairs receiving the blood. After the neglectful care Mom had been receiving, I was leaving nothing to chance. Abe came on the line to tell me that Mom had just been wheeled to the lab. As we were talking, the call waiting on my cell phone beeped. I asked Abe to hold on, so I could tell the caller I would phone back.

"This is the business office at Palmeros Community Hospital," a woman's voice said. "I've been authorized to tell you that Mrs. Helfant's Medicare coverage runs out today. If we do not receive a check for three thousand dollars within three working days, you will be asked to remove her from The Villa."

I stared at the phone in disbelief. At the very moment I was calling to be certain my mother was receiving blood transfusions to correct a life-threatening medical error that had been caused by a negligent physician, some bureaucrat was telling me to hand over three thousand dollars, or they would throw a seriously sick old woman out of their hospital. This could have been the stuff of Comedy Central if it were not so deadly serious. Had modern medicine really come to this?

"Do you know that while we're talking, my mother is receiving two units of blood at your hospital?"

"I'm sorry, sir," came the reply, "but we have our rules and regulations. Medicare…"

"The hell with your rules and regulations! Don't you people know, or care, that my mother is still a sick woman?"

"Sir, I have my instructions. If the check is not in our hands within three working days, your mother will have to leave our facility." She hung up.

Cursing the dial tone, I threw the phone on the bed and shouted a stream of expletives. Then I sat down and wrote Palmeros Hospital a check for three thousand dollars. Mom was no longer stable and until she stopped hemorrhaging, moving her to another facility would involve real risk. Once again, there seemed no choice but to comply with the system.

Two days and two additional transfusions later, Mom finally seemed to be out of danger. The hemorrhage had stopped on a lower dose of blood thinner, and the anemia was corrected. That evening, I was in the hospital parking lot, about to get into my car when someone called my name. It was Dr. James Ellis, an old friend from New York, and a gastroenterologist in the neighboring town of El Centro.

It was wonderful to see a familiar face. After telling Jim about Mom's illness and the problems with Doleman, I asked if he would agree to take over her case. All Mom needed, I said, was a nice doctor who would keep an eye on things until she completed her convalescence.

Jim dropped his eyes. "I know Doleman. He and his partner run the ICU at our hospital. To be honest, I can't afford to antagonize them. I depend on those guys for referrals. But I'll check around and see if I can find someone else to take care of your mother."

After two days of silence, I phoned Jim's office. He was unavailable. I left a message. Four calls and three days later, he picked up the phone.

"I called two people. One doesn't want to do it. He's afraid of offending Doleman too. The other doc is willing. Remember, you did not get the name from me."

By the next morning, Mom had a new doctor—a local family practitioner named Judith Croft. Jim had apprised her of Mom's blood clot problem. He had agreed with my treatment approach, and so did Dr. Croft. Mom had been on the lower dose of blood thinner for almost a week, and her blood tests had stabilized in the therapeutic range between one and a half and two times normal. There were no more signs of bleeding.

The following afternoon, Mom and I were engrossed in another crossword puzzle marathon when one of the nurses came in to give her medications. As Mom took them in hand, I noticed two unfamiliar pills. "What are the new drugs?" I asked, reluctant to play medical detective, but by now feeling that there was no choice.

"I don't know."

Abe avoided my gaze when I approached the nurses' station. "My mother's getting two new meds. Can you tell me what they are?" When he shrugged, I pointed to the chart rack.

"There's a written order not to let you look at your mother's chart," he said. Then he leaned over and whispered, "I'm going into the back room."

Abe withdrew, and feeling like Agent Mulder from *The X Files*, I rifled through the chart bin, while keeping an eye out for intruders. Finally, I located Mom's records and saw that one of the new drugs was thyroid hormone. The other was an antidepressant. Did Mom have a malfunctioning thyroid gland? Was she depressed? I flipped through the lab reports. No evidence of a thyroid problem. As for being depressed, Mom had become The Villa's daytime talk show host. All the nurses and orderlies adored her, and she seemed to be having the time of her life, reveling in the attention. These drugs not only were unnecessary, they had potentially serious side effects. Once again, I was going to have to talk with Mom's doctor.

I called Dr. Croft's office from the nurses' station, only to be greeted by an answering machine. "This is Dr. Croft. I'm away on vacation for the next two weeks. If you have an urgent problem, please go to the Palmeros Community Hospital Emergency Room at…"

My first reaction was that there must be some mistake. I had met with Dr. Croft three days ago, when she agreed to take over Mom's care. Never did she mention a two-week vacation.

But by now, nothing surprised me. I managed to find out the name of the doctor covering for Croft and got him on the phone. "Frankly," he said, "Dr. Croft didn't tell me a thing about your mother. If she gets sick,

I'll get involved. Otherwise, you'll have to wait for Croft to get back. Sorry, but I've got to run."

Finally, I decided to let it go. Mom was scheduled for discharge in a week, and neither the thyroid medication nor the antidepressant would have begun to take effect before then. When Mom finally got home, I would simply stop both drugs.

∞

August 7th was Mom's eighty-seventh birthday, and Abe and the nurses decided to throw her a party. The birthday girl spent hours primping for the occasion. With her snow-white hair newly permed, her face in full makeup mode, and fashionably bedecked in her most floral robe, Mom made a triumphant entrance into the dining room—adorned with balloons and streamers—to the applause of her staff pals. Seated at the head of the table, she beamed as we sang "Happy Birthday," blew out the candles with a flourish, and cut the cake. Mom was delighted by a bevy of presents: a bouquet of roses, a bottle of her favorite perfume, and a fat new book of *New York Times* crossword puzzles. Rising from the far side of the table and holding up a glass of grape juice, Abe toasted Mom.

"Annie, you could hardly walk when you first came here, and now…you're looking mighty fine, baby! Here's to another eighty-seven years."

Everyone rose and lifted their glasses in a joyous salute. "To Annie!" Beaming, Mom took a sip of her juice, and said, "Thank you for being so wonderful to me. I love every one of you. Now please sit down and eat your cake!"

∞

After the party, I suggested a quiet dinner on The Villa patio. En route, Mom asked why everyone had been so laudatory at her party. "After all, reaching eighty-seven is not that big a deal."

"It was a lot more than that. They remember how frail you were when you first came to The Villa. Then, they saw how you rallied after the hemorrhage. You never wavered. Just kept fighting. Everyone here admires your courage."

"You mean they think I'm one tough cookie?"

During dinner, Mom's mood shifted. Absently picking at her food, she gazed toward a cluster of palm trees shading a sprawl of multicolored flowers. At the top of a nearby hill, a cottontail rabbit hurried off into the underbrush.

"You know, I'd forgotten how beautiful the world is. I'm glad God decided to let me enjoy it a while longer."

Mom looked skyward. Sifting through luminous clouds, the slowly setting sun cast a pink glow over the scene.

"Remember when I first came out of the coma and I told you that God was keeping an eye on me?" she asked.

"Yup."

"Well, He always has."

"Of course."

"No, you don't understand." Mom took my hand in hers. "I'm going to let you in on a secret. When I was, you know, in that coma, I had the feeling that God was talking to me."

"Really? What did He say?"

"He said I was going to be okay. And later, with that hemorrhage business, I was feeling a whole lot sicker than I let on. One night, I thought I might be dying."

"Why didn't you say anything?"

"It seemed like everyone was doing whatever they could for me, and I didn't want to be a bother. But I did talk to God. I asked Him if I was dying. He assured me that He'd see me through that ordeal too. That's when I told you I wasn't concerned, and that nothing was going to stop me from going home."

Suddenly, a stern look came over Mom's face. "Promise that you won't say a word about this to anyone. I don't want people to think I've become a crazy old woman."

"Scout's honor," I said, smiling.

∞

Three days later, amid cries of "Good luck, Annie," Mom and I exited the corridors of The Villa, and walked out of Palmeros Community Hospital. As she approached the waiting taxi, Mom looked back to The Villa. "The people here were all so lovely," she said, "but it's a shame I never met my doctors."

I didn't say a word.

∞

In the years that followed her illness, Mom underwent profound changes. She became more reflective and serene, quietly savoring the landscapes that surrounded her. She abandoned her lifelong passion for politics, stopped watching CNN and C-SPAN, and instead immersed herself in books about Judaism by authors like Martin Buber and Abraham Joshua Heschel.

Whenever I would bring up one of the latest issues dominating the front pages of the newspapers, Mom no longer expressed interest, preferring to talk about religious matters. Increasingly, she was coming to embrace the ancient Hebrew view of eternity.

"I don't believe there's such a thing as heaven or hell. What I see is an exquisite reuniting with God." When I expressed surprise, Mom confided that she had become engaged in an ongoing dialogue with the Almighty.

Crossword puzzles remained our favorite pastime, and Mom's level of engagement and sharpness was as acute as ever. But as time passed, she became more withdrawn. One day, I asked her about it.

My mother smiled at me knowingly. "Concerned about your Mom, darling son? Don't worry. That heat stroke didn't cause any brain damage, and I haven't gotten senile either. The woes of the world still concern me. It's just that they no longer preoccupy me." Mom gave my hand a conspiratorial squeeze. "Since my illness, I've discovered more valuable ways to spend the time God has given me. Of course, I'm ready to go whenever He calls."

Mom looked outside her living room window. "The wonder of nature is so enthralling. Perhaps in some way, beauty will save the world."

Getting misty, Mom shifted her gaze to me. "Of all my blessings, I treasure my precious family most—you and your sister, my three darling grandchildren. I have so much to live for."

"Well, your family loves having you around, and we hope you stay with us for a long time."

Mom leaned over and kissed my cheek. "When my time comes, it will be nice to know that I'll live on in my children and grandchildren."

Mom died in her sleep three years later at the age of ninety.

Wall Street Willie

"What is the end of avarice and ambition,
of the pursuit of wealth, of power?"
—Adam Smith

I long ago learned that powerful people often use bluster and bombast to conceal their fears. But nothing could have prepared me for the human tornado who had just blown into my office.

Approaching my desk, he slowly took in the room. "Nice setup you have here, Doc. Those diplomas are very impressive."

"Thank you," I said.

Putting his hands on his generous hips, he threw back his shoulders and looked at me quizzically.

"Please have a seat," I said, pointing to an adjacent chair.

"Don't you know who I am?" he asked.

"Apart from your name, I have no idea."

"I thought all you doctors read *The Wall Street Journal*."

"*The New England Journal*'s more my speed."

"Okay, Doc, here's the deal. You think my name's Will Piersall, but ever since that article in the *Journal* last year, I've been rechristened Wall Street Willie. They call me a tycoon, because I'm a really rich son of a bitch."

Letting out a gleeful guffaw, Will deposited himself into the chair.

"What brings you to see me?" I asked.

"I'm told that you're the guy to see about bum tickers," Will said, leaning back in his rumpled Armani suit, pink shirt, and a Sulka tie that hung unceremoniously over his ample belly. A shiny bald pate accentuated his pudgy face and unblinking owlish eyes.

"Look. Since we're going to be friends, there's something you should know about me," he said.

"What's that?"

"I always take very good care of my friends. Now maybe you better begin checking me out."

Will had a history of diabetes and high blood pressure. That was not surprising, because in susceptible people, obesity commonly causes or worsens both of these disorders. Eighty to 90 percent of adult diabetics are obese.

Diabetic patients are unable to metabolize sugar properly, either because of an insufficient production of insulin, as in Type 1 diabetes, or because they do not respond to insulin properly, as in Type 2 diabetes. The latter condition, referred to as insulin resistance, occurs primarily in adults. Fully 80 percent of patients with this disorder die of cardiovascular diseases.

High blood pressure, also called hypertension, has dire consequences as well. The American Heart Association has called it the silent killer, because without causing symptoms itself, hypertension frequently gives rise to lethal diseases such as heart attacks and strokes. The obesity epidemic in the United States has led to a dramatic increase in the prevalence of diabetes and hypertension. Some studies have concluded that as many as 40 percent of Americans have elevated blood pressure.

Diabetes and hypertension are themselves perilous diseases, but in recent years, we have learned that they are the tip of an iceberg of abnormalities that have been grouped under the name metabolic syndrome. In addition to diabetes and hypertension, these patients have a uniquely malevolent combination of lipid abnormalities that markedly accelerate the development of atherosclerosis, heart attacks, and strokes: high triglyceride levels, low HDL ("good" cholesterol), and a particularly dense and dangerous form of LDL ("bad" cholesterol). They also have an increased tendency to form blood clots. More than three million Americans are estimated to have the metabolic syndrome, and untreated, their life expectancy is reduced by more than a third.

Since obesity is the common denominator, weight reduction and simple lifestyle changes can reverse many of these life-threatening abnormalities. The Framingham Heart Study found that as weight rises and falls, so too do blood pressure and blood sugar. Unfortunately, few heed the warning. Only 7 percent of patients with the metabolic syndrome are able to bring cardiac risk factors to desired levels. Arguably, this is the most important health care problem in the United States.

But now was not the time to raise diet and lifestyle issues with Wall Street Willie. First, I had to focus on whether or not he was in any danger. Were his risk factors already causing cardiac symptoms?

"Are you experiencing chest discomfort of any kind?"

Shifting uneasily in his chair, Will said, "I'd like to call you Dick, unless you have a problem with that."

"No problem at all. What about chest discomfort?"

"I'm a golf nut, Dick," he said, "and most of my deals are done on the course. A round of golf is a great way to size up a guy. When there's money riding on the game, you can see how he performs under stress. There he is standing over a three-foot putt with a couple grand on the line. You're giving him shit to amp up the pressure. How bad does he want to win? Will he choke? Does he cheat?"

"Do you?"

Will threw back his head and let out a hearty cackle, sending his belly reverberating. "All the time, Dick. All the time."

"You still haven't answered my…"

"I'm getting to that," he said.

Getting straight answers from this Wall Street Willie was more difficult than trying to catch water in a sieve. To cut through his outsized verbal smokescreen, I would have to listen with particular care, not only to what he said, but also to how he said it, and to be alert to unspoken clues such as changes in eye contact and body posture. Getting to the root of any patient's problem calls for concentration and focus, but in this case, it was indispensable to understanding this audacious patient's heart.

"Last week," Will continued, "I had three underwriters in from Boston. These geeks are more like undertakers than underwriters, but I need them to finance this huge megadeal I'm putting together. It's one of the biggest buyouts I've ever done. Anyway, I figure I'll soften them up a little, by taking them out for a round at the club. If you remember, it was really hot and humid last week, but we go out and everything is proceeding as planned." Suddenly, Will's eyes dropped to the floor.

"What happened?"

"It was nothing really," he mumbled. "I'm on the first tee, taking a couple of practice swings…"

"And?"

"And, I got this little squeezy sensation. Only lasted a minute or two."

"Where did you feel it?"

"Dick, I'm telling you, it was nothing," Will said, while making a fist with his left hand and putting it over the center of his chest.

I sprang to attention. Will had silently supplied a crucial clue. A fist pressed over a patient's chest is a classic sign that the symptom is cardiac in origin. It is the equivalent of angina pectoris, the chest pain that results from one or more blocked coronary arteries supplying blood to the heart.

"Did you feel anything else?"

"A little short of breath, but hell, you'd be breathing hard too if you had to lug this tub of blubber around in all that heat. It was just too damn hot to play golf."

When shortness of breath accompanies the squeezing chest discomfort of angina pectoris, it is disturbing. After a portion of a patient's heart muscle becomes oxygen deprived, it stops contracting within seconds. If the blood supply is restored before damage (a heart attack) occurs, the area resumes normal function. When shortness of breath occurs during an episode of angina pectoris, it indicates that a large part of the heart has been affected, and that serious cardiac dysfunction has resulted. My concern was growing.

"Did you experience light-headedness or dizziness?"

"Maybe a touch, but when I sat down for a few minutes, pretending to recalculate the bet, it went away. After that, we played nine holes, and I was fine. Won the bet too. Five grand!"

"Don't you usually play the full eighteen holes?"

"Yes, but like I keep telling you, it was hot as blazes out there, and after the front nine, I was exhausted."

"How did you…"

"Dick, it's time to cut to the chase. The only reason I came here today was to convince those Boston bozos that there's nothing wrong with me. After that shit on the first tee, they're all uptight, asking a bunch of questions about my health, and unless I satisfy them, the deal is off. So, my friend, I need you to give me a clean bill of good housekeeping."

"What do you mean?"

"I mean write me a nice little note on your official Heart Institute stationery giving my heart a triple-A rating, and send me a bill for whatever. Believe me, I'll make it worth your while."

Giving Will a clean bill of health might be good for his bank account, and perhaps mine too, but it could prove disastrous for his health. Light-headedness during an attack of anginal chest pain suggests that either the temporarily dysfunctional heart is not pumping sufficient blood to the brain, or that the oxygen-starved area has caused a brief cardiac rhythm disturbance. Both are ominous indications of possibilities yet to come. Most heart attack fatalities result from sudden, catastrophic rhythm abnormalities that occur before a patient can reach the hospital.

Will tried to dismiss his symptoms on the first tee because he was able to play the rest of the round, but that is a common occurrence in patients with anginal chest discomfort. All golfers know that the stress is highest before they hit the first tee shot. After that, they become more relaxed.

Stress creates a domino effect that leads to angina pectoris. The blood pressure rises, putting a strain on the heart that increases its need for oxygen. At the same time, the coronary arteries constrict. When this occurs in already blocked vessels, blood flow to the heart is reduced at precisely the time that it needs to be enhanced.

In addition, stress activates factors in the blood that form clots. Usually, when the stress eases, these factors normalize and the immediate threat recedes. Often, the clots dissolve. But once set in motion, the combination of blood vessel constriction and increased clot activation can also create an irreversible cascade of events culminating in a blocked-off artery and a heart attack.

"Will, I'd love to be able to write that note for you, but..."

Will responded by opening his shirt and exposing his hairy chest. "Look Dick, just stick your stethoscope here, and give me the note."

"Will, your symptoms strongly suggest a serious heart problem. I need to do a complete evaluation. At that point, we can sit down and discuss the problem."

The physical examination can reveal invaluable information about the extent of a patient's cardiovascular disease. In a patient with diabetes and hypertension, the eyes are mirrors of his vascular system. The extent of vascular abnormalities seen in the retina of diabetics correlates with the overall severity of their vascular disease, and their prognosis. The same is true of patients with high blood pressure.

An evaluation of the carotid arteries in the neck, which supply blood to the brain, is also vital. A reduced pulse in either vessel is a sign of blockage, as are abnormal sounds of blood turbulence (bruits) heard through a stethoscope. A partial carotid artery blockage increases the risk of a life-threatening stroke.

Bruits can be detected in other areas as well, such as the kidney and groin arteries. The absence of the normal pulses in the feet is another indication of widespread vascular disease.

"Come on, Dick. Are you worried I might sue if you don't give me a complete evaluation?" Will said, as he finished unbuttoning his shirt. "Forget it. You don't have anything like the money it would take to make it worth my while, and neither does your insurance company."

"Will, this isn't about money. If you won't let me evaluate you properly, the only option is for you to find another cardiologist."

"Great word you used there, Dick."

"What word was that?"

"Option. I'm an options trader. I love options."

"Before I can give you any options, we need to do the physical and get the test results. I'm sure you wouldn't consider buying a company without knowing every detail about its strengths and weaknesses."

Will scratched his nose and seemed to be pondering my proposal. Finally, he leaned on his elbow and pointed a finger at me. "Got a deal for you, Dick. I'll agree to come back and do all that stuff. But now, you check my heart out, and give me that note. I got a meeting in twenty minutes."

Leaning back in his chair, Will bared his chest.

"Sorry, but I cannot write notes without knowing what's going on. Frankly, I'm concerned that you may not be stable."

"Dick, my life is never stable, and I like it that way. Living on the edge, making outrageous bets, pulling off deals that the so-called pundits think are impossible is what I do."

"Will, this is not about a deal; it's about your life! I'm sure you'd agree that there's never a reason to take unnecessary risks."

Will began rebuttoning his shirt.

"Risk. There's another great word. Last year I fired my accountant. Want to know why? Because my tax returns hadn't been audited in three years. You're probably thinking, 'Isn't that good?' The answer is, not for me because I see my IRS return as an opening bid. When the feds don't audit me, it means my accountant's been too gutless to take them on.

"The point is, I handle risk better than anyone on the planet. That's why I'm the best at what I do," Will said, while straightening his tie.

"Will, none of that has anything to do with what I'm talking about."

"Don't insult my intelligence, Dick. I know damn well what you're talking about. In fifteen minutes, I'm going to wave a magic wand and blow so much bullshit at those Boston bean counters that they'll think King Midas is behind this deal. But I can't have them questioning *anything*, particularly about my health. Now, is that hard to understand?"

"Of course not, but I wouldn't be doing my job if I didn't tell you what I think. It's your choice."

"Always is." Will rose. "I'm out of here, Dick. You're a decent, devoted guy. Just send that little note to my office, and maybe I'll invite you out to the club for a round of golf. Introduce you to some people who can do you a hell of a lot of good. If you want to lay your hands on some real money for your research, you should be cultivating fat cats like me, not begging for crumbs at the NIH."

"After we check you out," I said smiling.

"I'm expecting that note in tomorrow's mail. Don't disappoint me," Will said as he closed the door behind him.

∞

I did not send the note, and Will never called. Two months later, my secretary buzzed the intercom. Will was calling from Hilton Head Island.

"Got an interesting story for you, Dick," he began, as though we'd just chatted the day before. "You don't know this, but one of my companies owns half this island. I come here all the time. Great golf courses, terrific food. Anyway, last night I was at the villa, having a fabulous time with this amazing girl. You know, cozy fire, Dom Perignon, full moon, crashing waves, Sinatra in the background—the whole routine. We're getting it on, and all of a sudden, that squeezing thing started. It felt like a fucking elephant was standing on my chest. I couldn't breathe, couldn't even move. The girl went nuts trying to get me off her. I swear, I thought she was going to have a heart attack too. Are you following me so far?"

"Sure am," I said, trying to keep calm.

"Anyway, after the chest pain eased off, we both settled down. Chilled for maybe half an hour, had a couple glasses of Dom, checked out the moon shining on the bay. It was a beautiful night. Then we started where we left off, and, Dick, I'm telling you, it was the greatest sex of my life. Slept like a baby the rest of the night, and woke up feeling like a million, no, a billion bucks."

My first instinct was to say, "You macho idiot, get yourself to the nearest hospital. Now!" But I stopped myself. Heart attacks commonly occur during sexual intercourse, and despite his bravado, I knew Will called because he was frightened, so I proceeded slowly.

"How long did the chest pain last?"

"I don't know. Maybe fifteen or twenty minutes."

Typical anginal chest pain lasts five to fifteen minutes. When the pain continues for more than a half hour, the probability of its being a heart attack increases. Will had been moments from a coronary.

"It must have been pretty scary."

"A little, to be honest. But you know, us tough guys just got to get up and get back on the horse." A roar of laughter blared through the phone.

There were a host of things that could be done to decrease the likelihood of blood clots forming in Will's coronary arteries, while stabilizing the blockages. The approach is to attack on all fronts: Prevent clots with anticoagulants. Alleviate blood vessel spasm with vasodilator drugs. Decrease cardiac stress by lowering the blood pressure. Decrease the cholesterol levels. Reduce inflammation. And if medications fail, bring in the heavy artillery: balloon dilatation or coronary bypass surgery. How could I get this man to listen, and stop channeling everything through the invincible Wall Street Willie façade? Where was Will Piersall, whose life was in jeopardy?

"Will, you were lucky last night, but you're playing Russian roulette with your life. You need medical attention right away."

"I figured you might say something like that. I'll have my secretary make an appointment with you when I get back to town."

"Next time, you may not be so lucky."

"I've always been lucky, and I intend to stay that way. Have a good day, my friend."

∞

A week later, my pager went off during rounds. It was the emergency room. "We need you down here right away."

"What's going on?"

"One of your patients was just brought in by ambulance."

"Who is it?"

"We don't have his records. Seems he was starting to play a round of golf, and had severe chest pains."

"I'll be right down."

"I should warn you, it doesn't look good."

When I got to the ER, it was 11:15 a.m., and things were quiet, except for a blur of activity on the far side of the nurses' station. Kenny, one of the interns, came over as I approached the group.

"The guy's had a massive coronary. I think he may be going into shock."

"What are his vital signs?"

"When he came in, his blood pressure was 120 over 90. Now, it's 100 over 70. Here's the electrocardiogram. Man, it's ugly."

"I'd like to see the patient first."

Sitting up on a gurney, Will smiled sheepishly, and in a weak voice, whispered, "When you said I was playing Russian roulette, you never told me how many bullets were in the chamber, Dick."

"Well, maybe it bounced off that hard head of yours without doing too much damage," I said, squeezing my patient's hand. Will's fleshy face was dusky and mottled with blue and red blotches, all signs of a failing circulation. But his eyes looked clear, and he seemed amazingly alert.

"What happened?" I asked, while beginning my physical exam.

"This guy needs me to help him underwrite a deal, so knowing that I love golf, he suggests we play a round on his course. He belongs to the Merion Golf Club, one of the country's great courses, so…"

"Will, time is critically important."

"Okay," Will said. "I'm setting up the bet in the locker room, when a wave of nausea comes over me. It was weird, because I didn't eat much breakfast. But after a few minutes, it goes away, and we go out to the first tee, and I'm in the middle of a practice swing, when I feel nauseous again. Then this unbelievable pressure hits me, just like at Hilton Head, like that fucking elephant was back on my chest. I went kind of wobbly. Couldn't feel my legs. Sweat was pouring out of me, and even though it was hot out there, I was freezing. I knew if I didn't sit down, I was going to faint." Will closed his eyes and fell back on the gurney.

"The guy helped me to the bench, and called 911. I don't know if I passed out or what, but the next thing I knew, they were putting me into an ambulance. Thank God they gave me that morphine. The pain was crushing the life out of me."

I put my stethoscope to Will's chest. His heart was racing at 150 beats per minute—about twice normal. The heart sounds were diminished due to weakened contractions, and the crackling noises at the bases of his lungs signaled the beginning of heart failure.

If more than 40 percent of the heart is damaged, the remaining muscle cannot adequately perform the task of pumping blood to meet the body's needs. In Will's case, the physical examination strongly suggested that the portion under siege exceeded 40 percent.

But there was still hope that things could be turned around. While the blood clot that blocked Will's coronary artery caused his heart attack, the portion of his heart being starved of oxygen and nutrients had not yet been irrevocably damaged. If left untreated, it would slowly die over a period of a few hours. We had a precious window of opportunity to open the clogged vessel and save a portion of the jeopardized area. Will's life depended on how quickly and completely we could act.

I asked Kenny for the electrocardiogram and blood work, and had him alert the cardiac catheterization lab to prepare for an emergency procedure.

The electrocardiogram confirmed the severity of Will's heart attack. The ST segment of the EKG, the key indicator of damage, was off the charts. But there was an important bit of good news. The portion of the electrocardiogram called the Q wave had not yet formed. The presence of Q waves indicates that irreversible muscle damage has already occurred. There was still time to salvage a major portion of Will's threatened heart muscle. But blood tests called cardiac troponin and CK-MB, also indicators of irreversible damage, were already slightly elevated.

For a patient in the throes of a heart attack, the best way to minimize the damage is to dilate the occluded coronary artery with a balloon-tipped catheter, a procedure called a coronary angioplasty. The deflated balloon is threaded from an artery in the groin into the area of the blockage. When inflated, it shoves the clot aside, opening the artery. A successful dilatation procedure decreases the size of a heart attack, improves survival rates, and significantly decreases the chances of the patient's having either another attack or a stroke.

Everything now depended on opening Will's blocked artery before the damage became irrevocable. Removing my stethoscope, I asked Will the critical question.

"When did your symptoms begin?"

Will looked at the emergency room clock. "About two and a half hours ago. Why?"

"You're having a coronary, and it's a big one. We need to get you to the lab immediately for an angiogram. It will give us x-ray pictures of your coronary arteries, so we'll know how many blockages you have and where they're located. After that, the chances are we'll want to do a balloon angioplasty."

"What's the deal with the balloon job?"

"A catheter is threaded into an artery in the groin up to the blocked area, and the artery is opened up with a balloon."

"Is that my best option?"

"Yes. After that, we'll go from there."

Kenny was giving me the high sign from the nurses' station. The catheterization lab was ready for our patient.

"It's time to get you up to the lab."

"Tell me the downside of the balloon, Dick. Give me worst case."

"Let's go," I answered. "I'll tell you on the way."

As Will's gurney sped along the hospital corridors en route to the catheterization lab, he was still asking questions.

"If you can't do the balloon job, are we talking about a bypass operation?"

"If the occluded part of the artery is inaccessible, or if it's filled with calcium and the balloon can't crack it open, we'll have to consider a bypass."

"Am I awake during the balloon job?" he asked as we entered the laboratory.

"Yes. We'll give you a local anesthetic to numb the groin area. If you like, you can watch the entire procedure on one of the TV monitors."

Will leaned back to get a better look at the TV screens. "Okay, Dick, let's do it. But if I need the bypass option, you talk to me about it beforehand. Deal?"

"Deal," I said.

∞

Most patients gratefully accept a mild sedative and a painkiller while an angiogram is being done. It allows them to relax while remaining awake, although many doze off during the procedure. Will refused all medicines, and after each angiogram was taken, he wanted to know what it showed.

The angiograms revealed that the vessel called the left anterior descending artery, or LAD, supplying the major portion of the heart muscle, was ninety-eight percent blocked by a fresh blood clot. Only a trickle of blood seeped through the obstructed area. While the other arteries had minor blockages, none harbored clots, or reduced blood flow to the heart.

"What's the plan?" Will asked.

"We need to go after the clot that's causing the heart attack. Once we dilate it open, the area…"

"What about those other blockages?"

"They are not causing any problems right now. The best way to deal with them is to reduce your coronary risk factors and use anticoagulants to reduce the risk of future clots."

"Can't you open up those suckers too? I don't want to be sitting on a time bomb waiting for another heart attack."

"Ballooning those blockages will not prevent you from having another heart attack."

"Why not? If there are no more blockages, then I'll be home free, and my worries will be over."

While Will's question was understandable, it flew in the face of everything that was known about optimal treatment of patients in his situation. Contrary to popular belief, heart attacks are *not* caused by large cholesterol buildups, but by small fatty accumulations prone to develop inflammation. The vulnerable buildups are filled with fatty cholesterol and covered by thin caps, while the larger buildups contain less fat and have thicker caps. At least 75 percent of heart attacks are caused by the rupture of the seemingly inconsequential cholesterol buildups.

"Will, the best way to prevent you from getting another heart attack is not by ballooning those blockages, but by lowering your blood sugar and cholesterol levels, getting your blood pressure into the normal range, and giving you drugs that will make it more difficult for blood clots to form in your arteries."

"I don't like your plan. It's not aggressive enough. Why not take the bull by the horns and balloon everything in sight?"

"Because a huge amount of research has shown that the plan I want to follow is the most effective way to decrease your risk. It will reduce *all* the vulnerable cholesterol buildups in your coronary arteries, not just the larger ones."

"I still can't understand why…"

"Will, please believe me. We are going to be very aggressive here. Even if we ballooned everything in sight, your risk of a having another heart attack would remain high. But hitting those risk factors of yours hard will reduce the chances by 80 percent, if not more."

"I sure hope you know what you're doing."

The balloon dilatation of the LAD went without a hitch. The massive ST segment elevations on Will's electrocardiogram soon returned to normal, and all indications were that the amount of heart muscle damage would be small. I started Will on medications to prevent further clots and others to lower his cholesterol, blood pressure, and blood sugar levels. Under close observation in the coronary care unit, he had no symptoms of chest discomfort or shortness of breath. An echocardiogram confirmed that his cardiac function had improved dramatically. Will was making a rapid recovery from his life-threatening heart attack.

But the ordeal had taken a toll on him. Over the next several days, Will's once grandiose mien dulled, and his arrogance morphed into inertia. When I asked how he was feeling, he displayed none of his usual bluster. A growing stack of unopened papers, letters, and a pile of *Wall Street*

*Journal*s accumulated on his night table. On the day of his scheduled discharge, I went alone to see Will.

"Everything looks good," I said. "You really dodged a bullet. Not many people win at Russian roulette when the bullet's in the chamber."

"I guess so," Will said woodenly. "You did a wonderful job, Dick, and I thank you."

I looked into Will's eyes, trying to get a sense of what lay behind this new persona. Bleary and unfocused, they betrayed nothing.

Was it our difficult discussion in the catheterization laboratory? Although he had not brought it up again, perhaps Will was preoccupied by the widespread abnormalities that had been seen on his angiogram studies. Had he become obsessed by the thought that an uncertain future now faced him? Did the once invulnerable Wall Street Willie fear that his life now hinged on the whim of a cholesterol deposit becoming inflamed resulting in a second, perhaps fatal heart attack? I had known many proud and powerful men who succumbed to feelings of shame, humiliation, and despondency in the aftermath of an illness. Their ordeal left them seeing themselves as fatally flawed beings, no longer masters of the realm.

"You've responded beautifully to the medications we began in the coronary care unit. Your blood pressure and cholesterol levels have both normalized."

The jowls on Will's fleshy face sagged as he shook his head. "I know that," he said.

"If we are vigilant about keeping your risk factors under control, and you stay on a solid diabetic diet and an exercise program, the chances of another heart attack will be substantially reduced."

Will put his hands to his forehead as if to contain a hidden pain. "Jesus, Dick. Don't you think I know that?"

"Then what is it, Will?"

"A lot of things have become clear to me these last few days. Do you know 'the rule of the fool'?"

"Can't say that I do."

"In every game, there's a fool, and when you play, the first thing you have to do is figure out who it is. If you can't find the fool, then the fool is you."

"I don't get the point."

"Remember what I said about the similarities between the work you and I do? Well, there's one big difference. What you do affects people's lives. What I've been doing affects nothing. I've never given a damn about the money. It was all about winning. When you win, a life is saved. When I win, a bunch of numbers move from one side of a ledger to another. In the game of life, I've been the fool."

"Will, you've been through a nightmare, and right now you're feeling vulnerable. It's common for someone whose life has been threatened. You need to heal emotionally as well as physically, and it takes time. Be patient with yourself."

"Whatever you say, Dick."

∞

When Will returned for an office visit a week later, dark sunglasses hid his eyes, and white stubble covered his face. Shuffling silently into the exam room, he appeared to have aged twenty years.

During the physical, Will sat with his shoulders hunched, his head hanging to his chest as if asleep. My attempts to make small talk were ignored. The exam showed a normal blood pressure. His heart function was good, as were the electrocardiogram and blood work. After completing the exam, I asked him to come into the consultation room to talk.

"Will, you seem more depressed than you were in the hospital."

"I'm okay."

"Are you concerned that you're going to have another heart attack, or a stroke because we didn't balloon those other blockages?"

"It's not about any of that. I said I'm okay."

Will slumped into a ball as if he were collapsing into himself. The room was heavy with the weight of his gloom.

"From a medical standpoint, you're doing great. There's every reason to think that you've got a lot of life ahead of you."

"Right."

"If it's not your health that's made you so despondent, then tell me what's going on."

"What's going on is that I'm depressed, Dick. You would be too if you realized that your life had all been nothing but a pile of crap."

"Don't you help people when you make money for them?" I said, straining to find something encouraging to say.

"Help people? Surely you jest. Look, Dick. You can put all the lipstick you want on a pig, but at the end of the day, it's still a pig. I screwed those dumb motherfuckers every chance I got, and enjoyed every minute of it. My life has really been exemplary: working eighty-hour weeks, doing deals, chasing babes, and greasing the palms of slimeball politicians, while totally ignoring my family. And you know what that *Wall Street Journal* article called me? 'The personification of the American Dream!'

"I'm in a deep, dark place, and the last thing I need to hear is a bunch of bullshit about the wonderful way I've spent my life. For me, it was one big amusement park. I played all the games, made all the rules, and won all the prizes. It was about the thrill of the ride, the brass ring, the danger of losing it all on one roll of the dice. Now, that guy is dead. There should be a new headline in *The Wall Street Journal:* 'Wall Street Willie dies doing a deal on the Merion Golf Course.'"

"Didn't you tell me a while ago that after a disaster, you have to pick yourself up and…"

"…start all over again? That's the point. I can't do it anymore because I'm not Wall Street Willie anymore. I feel like I've been gutted like a mackerel. There's nothing left inside."

"Then maybe it's time to think about who you'd like to become— maybe doing something different that would be more meaningful to you. A guy with your talents and resources can do anything."

Will dragged himself to his feet. "Spare me the dime store psychology, Dick. Nothing in this fucked-up world interests me. Frankly, I'd consider killing myself except that I'll be damned if I'm going to give those IRS boys the satisfaction of ripping off my corpse with their fucking death tax."

Of course, Will was right about my dime store psychology. While wanting to find something to say that he would find encouraging, I had long since concluded that Will was right about what his life had been.

∞

Two weeks later, Will returned. Although he remained symptom free while continuing to make an uneventful recovery from the heart attack, his scruffy beard and rumpled clothing gave him the look of a homeless person. After completing the evaluation, we again met in the consultation room.

After he sat down, Will asked for a piece of scratch paper, scribbled something, and handed it to me. The note had the name of a corporation with *AMEX* next to it. Puzzled, I looked at Will.

"Is this a stock tip?"

"It's a sure thing. You got a broker?" Without waiting for a reply, Will grabbed another piece of notepaper and wrote a name and number on it. "Call this guy. No questions. Just do it."

Will's attempt to assume his old air of authority was a caricature of his former self. The once rambling monologues were now terse sound bites, the once commanding voice a monotone, so lifeless and hollow that it sounded computer simulated. Will's pain was palpable.

"I'd like to talk about *you*, Will."

"There's nothing to talk about. Since my last visit, I've done zilch. Nada. Nothing. I haven't been to the office. Haven't even called in."

"What about that megadeal with the Boston bankers?"

"I walked away from it. What was the fucking point? Just the thought of shaving and putting on a suit and tie makes me want to puke. You know what they say about Wall Street? It's a street with a river at one end, and a graveyard at the other. That about sums it up for me."

"What about your family and your friends?"

"You want to know about my family and my friends? Okay, I'll tell you. My wife and I have been separated for years. My kids hate me, and I've got no friends. Any other questions?"

"Maybe a change of scene would do you some good. What about going down to Hilton Head? You love it there."

"Hilton Head is finito, kaput. I loved the trappings, not the place. At Hilton Head I was Wall Street Willie, Master of the Universe. Now, I'm a fat, used-up nothing. If I were a commodity, I'd tell you to sell me short. Soybean futures look better than mine."

"You told me the golf courses were…"

"Don't you get it? Golf was never about golf. It was like everything else: the rush of the deal du jour. Doing deals meant living on the edge, being the man, the center of wherever I happened to be. Without that, golf's a waste of time. Everything's a waste of time."

"Will, I'm concerned about you. Maybe it would help if you talked with someone. A professional."

"Me see a shrink? Are you serious? Fuck you!" Will rose from his chair, flung open the door, and slammed it on his way out.

He did not keep his next two appointments.

∞

Several weeks later, my secretary discovered a phone message on the office answering machine that had been recorded at four-thirty in the morning: "I decided to take your advice, so a week ago I hopped on my jet and came down to Hilton Head. Guess what? Your brilliant plan isn't working. I'm hunkered down like a dog in a hailstorm."

Five days later, Jean buzzed the intercom. Will was on the line. Picking up the phone, I prepared for the worst.

"Got an interesting story for you, Dick," he said in what sounded like a weak attempt to mimic Wall Street Willie.

"I'm all ears."

"I haven't slept a wink down here. Just tossing and turning and listening to the clock ticking my life away. Last night, I wound up turning on the TV. Kept flicking the remote up and down the gazillion channels, looking for something that would kill some time and take my mind off my shit. You have any idea how much crap is on the tube? Who watches that stuff? Anyway, I'm about to get cramps in my fingers, so I gave up, dragged myself out of bed, and went outside.

"There I was, butt naked, standing at the shoreline, staring into the blackness. For how long, I don't know. The darkness started lifting so slowly that I was barely aware of it."

There was a pause on the phone. When Will began to speak again, his voice was no longer flat and depressed.

"Then what happened was so fucking weird, I don't know how to say it without sounding like a hippie or a Jesus freak."

"Don't worry about how you sound. I'd like to hear more."

"Well, after the sun finally broke over the ocean, streams of white light shot through the cloud cover. When the rays hit the water, I swear to God, it looked like a billion diamonds dancing over the waves. Then, this flock of seagulls comes out of nowhere, races across the water in perfect formation, and soars straight into the horizon."

Despite himself, Will sounded like an awestruck child. Absent were the lifeless sound bites I had become used to since his heart attack. Will's words burst over the phone with animation and intensity.

"I breathed the salt air into my lungs. All of life seemed to be flowing through me. I know this will convince you that I've lost my total mind, but it felt like I was witnessing—no, that I was a part of—the miracle of existence."

"Incredible!"

"Incredible doesn't begin to describe it. No one would ever accuse me of being a true believer, but all I could think of at that moment was the Bible, where it says something like 'And the spirit of God moved upon the face of the waters. And God said, 'Let there be light. And there was light.'"

I stared dumbfounded at the receiver. Who was this person on the other end of the line? Could this really be Will Piersall? And, of all things, quoting from the Bible?

"So, before you have me put away," he quickly continued, "want to know what happened next?"

"I can't possibly imagine."

"I played golf."

"Golf?"

"That's right. There wasn't a soul out there. Just me, the course, and the little white ball."

"That must have been different. How did it feel?"

"Dick, it was more magnificent than the world's most beautiful woman. On the first tee shot, I'm always nervous, so I usually yank my driver back and wind up hitting a big, fat slice. Now, I come back nice and slow. The ball comes off the club perfectly. Then it begins to bend right. Another slice, same as always. But, instead of becoming crazed, I laughed out loud. I'm a hundred and fifty yards from the green, with two monster sand traps in front of me. The shot calls for a six-iron, my worst club. Ninety-nine times out of a hundred, I hit the damn thing into one of those traps, so lately I've been wimping out, hitting an eight-iron short of the green, and taking my bogey. But today, I figure, what the hell, and pull out the six."

"And?"

"The six-iron kisses the ball, lifts it off the grass, and sends the little white fucker flying over both traps, heading straight at the pin. Now, I'm looking at a twelve-foot putt for a birdie. I get behind the ball to see the contour of the green, and it's as though someone's drawn a line across the grass between the ball and the cup. All I have to do is roll it along the line and it falls in."

"Did you make it?"

"I've been playing that course for years and never birdied that first hole until today. After that, I could do no wrong. Kept hitting one pure shot after another. I've never played a round of golf alone in my life. Never played without having something on the line, never played without using a scorecard. And, Dick, none of that mattered! Went straight to fucking nirvana, and still haven't come back."

∞

About two months later, Will returned to the office. After weeks on a vegetarian diet and jogging along the beaches of Hilton Head, he had lost twenty-five pounds and the dark cloud that had been hanging over him. Clear-eyed and deeply tanned, my patient glowed with good health.

On his physical exam, Will's blood pressure was normal, his heartbeat strong. The blood tests showed that his cholesterol and blood sugar levels had decreased substantially. The most striking change was on his EKG. It showed no evidence of a heart attack. In fact, Will's heart had healed so completely that the tracing looked almost normal.

"You are doing incredibly well on every level, Will," I said, after completing his evaluation. "Medically speaking, things couldn't be any better. You really are an amazing guy."

"Thanks, Dick. I've never felt any better. At Hilton Head, I felt healthy for the first time in my life. The place is beautiful, and these days I actually taste my food. It's like I've been sleepwalking through life, and that sunrise somehow woke me up. But being back here feels like crap. I just can't breathe the fucking air in this city. It stinks of gas and garbage. It's freaky having to inhale air that you can see. All this shit really got me thinking."

"About what?"

"We need to clean up our act, Dick, and I mean that literally. The planet is going down the tubes just as sure as I was when my fat ass was a breeding ground for diabetes, high blood pressure, and one motherfucker of a heart attack. I've been doing a lot of reading about pollution—how it affects the air, the drinking water, and even our food. It's deadly. We're killing ourselves, and no one gives a damn, or even knows about it. How many people know or care about the poisons, pesticides, and industrial waste that affect our health? We have to document all this stuff so we can produce scientific evidence that shows what's going on. Until then no one's going to wake up to what's happening. It's like a disease. Before you can treat it, you need to understand what's causing it. And once I get the facts, it'll be time to go into phase two: getting the powers-that-be to change their modus operandi. Make sense to you?"

"It makes a lot of sense, but how are you going to get those powers-that-be to listen and *do* something? A lot of them are going to line up against you."

"You've forgotten something, Dick. I may not be Wall Street Willie anymore, but I still know every corporate CEO worth knowing. I understand how they think, what they're about, and how to get their attention. Plus, I'm still a wealthy man, and in this wicked world of ours, money is access. Every political hack this side of D.C. will sell his soul for a contribution to his election fund."

"No more a very rich son of a bitch?"

"Touché," Will said with a laugh. "Tackling this problem is going to be the toughest thing I've ever done, but I'm up for it. I know how to use money to shake up the system and put people together, but now it'll be for something worthwhile."

"You really *have* been doing a lot of thinking, Will. Frankly, I never thought I'd see the day when you…"

"Became a human being? I told you a long time ago that we were a lot alike. It was a lie then, but now I'm going to make it true."

∞

A few months later, Will moved to Hilton Head Island. He called occasionally, to let me know about his health and the progress of his work in the then fledgling ecology movement. Continuing on the vegetarian diet and exercise program, he had no more cardiac symptoms.

Will threw his talents and resources into fostering collaborations between scientists across the country, funding studies that documented the effects of fossil fuel emissions, pesticides, and greenhouse gases on acid rain and global warming, as well as the effects of fecal and toxic waste dumping on our rivers, lakes, and streams. He provided seed money that stimulated research into the development of renewable energy.

Will became a one-man lobby, pressuring former corporate cronies, government bureaucrats, and politicians to adopt stricter fuel emission standards, and to enact safe air and water legislation. By cultivating relationships with the media, Will was able to help make the public more aware of the dangers that greenhouse gases imposed on their health. Gradually, his calls tapered off, but Will continued to send cards during the holidays. The last few contained pictures of him, together with his two adult children and their families.

One of his last Christmas cards has remained with me. It read, "New rule for an old fool: The fool wants everything and values nothing. The wise man wants nothing and values everything."

Emergency Emma

"Imagination frames events unknown in wild,
fantastic shapes of hideous ruin."
—Hannah More

The first time she waddled into my office, her two-hundred-and-forty-pound body precariously perched on spindly legs, I sensed that caring for Emma Jorgensen was going to be a challenge. After collapsing into an armchair, she began to tug on a shapeless green housedress in a vain attempt to rearrange herself. Panting and perspiring profusely, the thirty-eight-year-old woman's fear-filled eyes darted around the room as though she thought that at any minute, a monster might jump out and attack her from the shadows. Her behavior seemed all the more odd, since I was the fifth or sixth physician she had seen in the past year.

Swiping the sweat across her brow with an oversized forearm and pulling her mop of greasy red hair over both ears, she said, in a squeaky voice that seemed too small for her bulk, "I hope you can help me, Doctor. Those other doctors keep saying that my symptoms are all in my head."

"What seems to be bothering you, Emma?"

"Bothering me? My problems aren't just bothering me, they're killing me. If you don't do something to help me, I am going to die. I just know it."

"What kind of symptoms are you having?"

Heaving a huge sigh, Emma shifted uncomfortably in her chair. "I don't know where to begin," she said. "Whenever I try to explain my symptoms to a doctor, he just rolls his eyes and tells me it's nothing to worry about." Emma hunched over and began to well up.

I reached for the box of tissues on my desk and handed them to Emma. She grabbed a handful, dabbed her eyes, and looked at me expectantly.

By now, I too had become a bit disconcerted. New patients rarely unravel within minutes of our first meeting. I needed to calm this beleaguered woman, and find out what was going on.

"Let's figure out how we can help you. How about starting at the beginning?" I said. "What was your first symptom?"

"One night, about three years ago, I woke up with a pounding sensation in my chest. My heart was racing so fast, I thought it was going to jump out of my chest. Then I began to get nauseous and dizzy. I called Dr. Cahill, my family doctor who's also my gynecologist, and when I went in to see her the next day, she found a tumor in my tummy. She said I needed to have an operation to remove it."

"What did she find?"

"A cyst on my ovary. It was nothing serious, but after the operation, the pounding and the dizziness became more frequent, so she sent me to a neurologist."

"Why a neurologist?"

"I'd read an article that said the three most common symptoms of brain tumors were headaches, nausea, and dizziness, so I asked her to send me to a specialist. He did a bunch of scans and electrical tests, and said everything was okay. He prescribed a tranquilizer, but I knew *that* wasn't going to solve my problem."

"Did the tranquilizer help?"

"A little at first, but then my symptoms got worse. When the pounding started, in addition to becoming dizzy and nauseous, my hands would begin to tingle and become numb. After a while, the numbness spread to my face. The whole area around my mouth would lose all feeling, except for a wired tingling sensation. I was sure I going to have a stroke. That's when Dr. Cahill referred me to an ENT doctor."

"An ears, nose, and throat doctor?"

"That's right. She thought my dizziness might be due to an inner ear problem. He examined me and said he wasn't sure what was going on, but that I needed an operation to get to the bottom of it. But I was too scared. Besides, I still hadn't recovered from the ovary surgery, and my wounds weren't healing right, so my gynecologist said that I should wait before having another operation."

Emma's story made me wince. She had unwittingly fallen into the maze of modern medicine. Each specialist viewed her symptoms through the prism of his own specialty, ordered the inevitable battery of tests, and treated her with a pill or a procedure without having a diagnosis. Medications are the fifth leading cause of preventable death in the United States.

"Why did she send you to me?"

"I told her I didn't think I had an inner ear problem, and that it had to be some kind of a heart condition. After all, how could an inner ear problem cause chest pains and shortness of breath?"

"Chest pain and shortness of breath? You didn't say anything about that."

"You said to begin at the beginning."

"Why don't you tell me about the chest discomfort? When did it start and what does it feel like?"

Emma put her plump little hands over her voluminous breasts. "It's not discomfort, Doctor," she said plaintively. "It's *pain*, the worst pain you can possibly imagine."

"Can you describe what it feels like?"

"What do you mean? I just did."

"Does it feel like a ripping, a tightness or a squeezing feeling, a heaviness, a…?"

"It feels like all of those things. When I get it, I start trembling and shaking. I feel like if it doesn't stop, I'm going to suffocate. Why are you asking me all these questions? Can't you just give me something?"

I explained that there are several causes for chest discomfort, and each has a telltale set of characteristics. For example, in patients with pleurisy, an inflammation of the lining of the lungs, pain occurs with deep breaths.

With an inflammation of the sac around the heart, called pericarditis, the pain increases when a patient lies down, and improves when they sit up and lean forward. In patients with blocked coronary arteries, the discomfort occurs during physical activity, like walking or climbing stairs. A bulging or tear in the aorta, the main artery in the body, also has characteristic features.

All these possibilities and more needed to be carefully explored by delving into the nuances of Emma's chest pain, as well as her palpitations and shortness of breath. But Emma seemed to have no interest in what I was saying. Whenever I tried to get a more precise description of her symptoms, she would burst into tears instead of providing an answer. I began to preface each question by explaining that to get to the root of her problem, it was essential to understand the exact nature of her chest pain, but Emma only issued the same whiny reply.

"You're going to tell me that I'm imagining the pains, Doctor. I know it."

Getting nowhere, I countered, "I'm asking these questions because I *do* take your symptoms seriously. Can you tell me when they began?"

Emma remembered that the precise moment was two years ago on the night her husband left her. According to Emma, she and her husband had been happily married for seventeen years.

"Then one day, he came home from work, sauntered into the living room, and announced that he'd fallen in love with some girl at work, and that our marriage was over. He said he was leaving me and moving in with her. All that time, I thought we had a wonderful relationship. Doctor, do you have any idea what something like that can do to a person?"

"It had to have been a terrible shock. You must have been devastated."

"To say the least. From then on, my life began to fall apart. I felt like an avalanche had fallen on me. I was lost, and had no one to turn to. None of our friends wanted to have anything to do with me. The whole thing was too embarrassing for them. I was lonely and frightened.

"Our house seemed so big without him there. At night, when it was quiet, every creak scared me. Food was the only thing that seemed to calm me down and make me feel better. I started to eat compulsively, especially at night. I've always been kind of heavyset, but I really ballooned up. One night, I woke up with terrible chest pains and shortness of breath. It felt just like a heart attack."

"Why did you feel so certain?"

"I know all about heart attacks, Doctor. I do volunteer work at a library, and I read all the health newsletters and look up a lot of things in medical books. Medicine has always fascinated me. I think I could have been a good doctor."

"What did the pain feel like?"

"Like someone punched me in the chest. I couldn't catch my breath, and my heart was racing out of control. I thought maybe if I had something to eat, it would relax me, so I wolfed down a pint of Ben and Jerry's cookie dough ice cream."

"Why didn't you call your doctor?"

"I did, but when I told her the story about my husband, she said the pain was nothing to worry about, that I was understandably upset because of what had happened."

"Did the food make things better or worse?"

Patients with peptic ulcers, acid reflux, or gallstones can get symptoms of chest discomfort. Food usually reduces the distress caused by ulcers and acid reflux, but it accentuates gallstone pain.

"It didn't seem to make any difference. My husband always kept a few bottles of vodka in the freezer, so I took a gulp, put a heating pad on my chest, and went to bed, hoping it would pass. After a while, I fell asleep, and when I woke up, it was morning and everything was back to normal."

"And that's when you went to see your gynecologist?"

"Yes. But the attacks are getting more and more frequent, and I'm really frightened."

Emma's description of her chest pains did not conform to any of the common causes of chest discomfort, but it was important not to overlook other serious possibilities. In patients with pleuritis, a rubbing sound can be heard with a stethoscope over the lungs during a deep inhalation. Pericarditis sounds like sandpaper being rubbed in synchrony with the heartbeat. Cardiac birth defects, diseases of the heart muscle, and valve abnormalities all provide telltale murmurs and other characteristic clues on the physical exam.

∞

"I haven't always been this big," Emma said as I struggled to wrap a blood pressure cuff around one of her massive arms, while fending off the fumes of her overpowering perfume. "In high school, I played center on the basketball team, and I was really good at track and field. You probably won't believe me, but I won a trophy in the javelin event. I loved sports."

"Did you have any physical problems when you were a teenager?"

"I made the college track team in my freshman year. During one of the meets, I threw the shot putt, and felt a terrible pain in my chest that knocked me to the ground. I was doubled over in agony. My heart was racing, and I couldn't catch my breath. One of the coaches ran over, and when I told him what was happening, he put me in a car and drove me to the school infirmary. The nurse examined me, gave me a pill, and sent me to the dorm to rest."

"Did she think anything was seriously wrong?"

"She didn't say anything, and I was too frightened to ask. The dorm was empty, and I was still in pain. I remember lying on my cot thinking that I was having a heart attack, and that I could die and no one would be there to help me. But even though I didn't die, I was sure that something serious happened."

"Why did you think that? Didn't it seem more likely that you simply strained a muscle in your chest making the throw?"

"Maybe that's the way you would have reacted, Doctor, but I was in agony and my heart was beating so hard that it felt like it was going to fly out of my chest. I was frightened, and felt certain that something serious had happened to me, and the nurse didn't want to tell me the truth. From then on, I knew things were never going to be the same. Needless to say,

I never played sports again. That's when my weight problems began. I've been pretty heavy over the years, but it's never been as bad as this."

By now, it had become clear that Emma's symptoms were psychological rather than medical. Despite her off-putting personality, the deep hurt that pervaded this woman's being moved me. The least I could do was provide her with a sympathetic ear to help ease her anguish, while reassuring her that nothing was wrong with her heart. Continuing to pursue Emma's history, I asked when her symptoms returned.

"Sometimes my heart would start to race and I'd get short of breath. That always scared me, but the chest pains never came back until my husband left."

Despite Emma's rapid pulse, her blood pressure was normal and her lungs sounded clear. On the cardiac exam, her heart impulse was normal, but when I placed the stethoscope under her left breast, the diagnosis immediately became obvious.

When Emma's heart contracted, a series of loud clicking sounds were audible. My patient had mitral valve prolapse.

The heart is divided into two sides, each having two chambers. The upper two are called atria, and the lower two are the ventricles. The right atrium and ventricle receive oxygen-depleted blood from the body and send it to the lungs, where its oxygen content is replenished. The left atrium then receives the rejuvenated blood, passing it along to the left ventricle. The powerful left ventricular chamber then pumps its contents back to the body.

The atria and ventricles are separated from each other by valves. The tricuspid valve is located on the right side of the heart, while the mitral valve resides on the left. When the mitral valve opens, blood exits the left atrium, travels through the valve, and enters the left ventricle. As the left ventricle begins to contract, the valve closes, preventing blood from moving backwards into the left atrium.

The mitral valve consists of two leaflets, or flaps, each in the shape of a parachute. Normally, both leaflets close in unison, but in patients with mitral valve prolapse, either the valve leaflets are too large, the chords that attach them to the heart are too long, or the connective tissue in the structure is more elastic than normal. In any case, one or both of them balloons, or flops—prolapsing into the left atrium. The characteristic click heard when one listens to the heart is caused by the sound of the valve leaflet prolapsing into the atrial chamber, much like a parachute in the wind.

Mitral valve prolapse is a relatively common condition, occurring in 2.5 to 5 percent of people in the United States. It is particularly prevalent in pre-menopausal women between the ages of fourteen and forty. There has been a considerable amount of speculation about how the valve abnormalities occur, but recent research has shown that there is a genetic predisposition for the syndrome. Between 20 and 50 percent of the relatives of mitral valve prolapse patients also have the syndrome.

Echocardiograms are a valuable means of evaluating patients with suspected mitral valve prolapse. The test confirms the diagnosis by demonstrating the prolapsing valve leaflets. In addition, the presence and severity of any blood leaking backwards across the valve from the ventricle to the atrium can also be detected. In Emma's case, I did not hear the telltale murmur suggesting the presence of a leak.

Patients with mitral valve prolapse often have symptoms that mimic serious illnesses like heart attacks and cardiac rhythm abnormalities, but in the vast majority of women, the condition is neither dangerous nor life threatening. Most of the close relatives of patients with mitral valve prolapse who demonstrate a floppy valve on echocardiography are completely free of symptoms.

The reason for the chest pains, palpitations, or shortness of breath that occur in some patients with mitral valve prolapse has never been understood. For want of a more scientific explanation, it has been hypothesized that their nervous systems are programmed to respond excessively to stress. For unknown reasons, they are triggered to react to unthreatening circumstances as though they were dangerous. This imbalance is called dysautonomia.

After putting my stethoscope in the pocket of my lab coat, I patted Emma gently on the shoulder. "I have wonderful news! Your symptoms are being caused by a benign condition called mitral valve prolapse."

"Mitral *what?*"

"One of the valves in your heart kind of flops backwards when your heart contracts. It's as if the valve is double-jointed, or more flexible than other valves. It bends more than usual. The important point is that in your case, the condition is harmless, and nothing to be concerned about."

"Something *is* wrong with my heart! I *knew* it!" Emma's face flushed with fear.

My relief at having found a benign cause for the symptoms that had been plaguing Emma was rapidly turning to disbelief.

"Emma, your heart is not..."

"Did you say the valve flops backwards?" Emma said in a voice so shrill that I thought it might shatter the windowpanes. "I don't understand what that means. How can a flopping valve cause all these terrible symptoms? It has to be a lot more serious than what you're saying. What are you hiding, Doctor?"

"I am not hiding *anything.* Heart valves are like rubber bands. When you stretch them, some are more elastic than others. Some mitral valve prolapse patients have symptoms identical to yours, although we don't know why. It seems to be caused by the way the nervous system..."

"My god. Are you telling me that I have a diseased heart *and* a disease in my nervous system?"

"No, Emma," I said in a soft voice. "I'm saying that your condition poses no threat to you. I know your symptoms are frightening, but I promise you are going live to a ripe old age."

"No threat to me? How can someone with a diseased heart and a nervous system that causes such symptoms possibly live to a ripe old age? Pardon me for saying this, Doctor, but I don't think you're being quite candid."

"Emma, please calm down. The reasons why the nervous system in some people with mitral valve prolapse causes chest pains, palpitations, and shortness of breath is not entirely clear, but one thing *is* clear. No matter how severe and frightening your symptoms are, they are *not* dangerous. You are *not* going to have a heart attack, and you are *not* going to die."

Emma wrapped her arms around her chest and burst into tears. "I don't know what's worse, being told I'm a head case, or that I have two terrible diseases."

"Emma, you do not have *any* diseases," I said, handing her a fistful of tissues, "You just happen to have a valve that varies slightly from normal. I'd like to get an electrocardiogram and an echocardiogram test. When I see you again next week, we'll start you on medication that should help to control your symptoms."

∽

The electrocardiogram was normal, and the echocardiogram showed the classic findings of mitral valve prolapse. But while the valve leaflets did flop into the left atrium during contraction of the left ventricle, there was no leakage of blood through the valve during the prolapse, and the valve structure itself was normal.

Rolling from side to side like a sailor on the high seas, Emma arrived at the office huffing and puffing. The scowl on her face told me I was in for another challenging session.

"The news is all good," I said, holding the echocardiogram report in my hand. "The valve is not leaking, and its structure is... "

"Since I saw you last week, Doctor, I've been doing a lot of reading," she said, oozing her vast frame into a wing chair. "You really didn't tell me the truth about the seriousness of my illness."

"Of course I did. There's nothing to hide."

Emma reached into her pocketbook, pulled out a notepad, and thumbed through it until she found the first page. "You neglected to tell me that patients with mitral valve prolapse can develop severe valve leaks and need heart surgery to fix it. In some patients, the valve can rupture..."

"In some patients that's true, but not in your case. *Your* valve is not leaking, and it is..."

"*And,* the most important thing you neglected to tell me is that patients with mitral valve prolapse can die suddenly and unexpectedly."

I looked into my patient's anxious eyes and reached out to her. "Emma, please listen carefully. The complications you've been reading about are rare, and they almost never happen in cases like yours."

"How can you say that, Doctor? I must have read a dozen articles about mitral valve prolapse, and every one of them talked at length about these terrible complications."

"It's not that simple. Mitral valve prolapse can be serious in rare instances, but in your case, the tests indicate that the condition is benign. The echo test shows that the valve structure is normal, and it's not leaking. Your electrocardiogram is normal. That makes the likelihood of…"

"I don't know what all that means. What I *do* know is that my symptoms are as serious as they can possibly be."

"In some cases, the prolapsing valve allows blood to leak back into the left atrial chamber, but the leak almost never becomes severe enough to require corrective surgery. And those patients have specific identifying characteristics. Most are men over the age of fifty, and in every instance have a telltale murmur that signals blood regurgitating through the leaking valve. You are not a fifty-year-old man, and more importantly, you don't have a leaking valve."

"But couldn't I develop a leak? Isn't it possible?"

"I suppose anything is possible, but the patients who develop severe leaks have valves that, unlike yours, are thickened and distorted."

"So finally you admit that it's possible? Why haven't you said anything about a heart attack?"

"People with mitral valve prolapse have as much chance of having a heart attack as those with normal valves. In a young woman like you, there is no reason to think that…"

"Doctor, I happen to know that patients who are afflicted with mitral valve prolapse disease die suddenly and unexpectedly. How can that be true if there's no risk of a heart attack?"

"Those cases are very rare, and the patients are older men who have a distinctive abnormality on their electrocardiogram that you do not have. Maybe I should have told you all this on your first visit, but I didn't want to confuse you with a lot of information that's irrelevant in your case."

"Perhaps you should have. Fortunately, I've done my homework, so I'm not confused."

∽

Experience has taught me that informed patients are better equipped to combat their illnesses. Those who ask questions usually want to understand their conditions as fully as possible, because the information decreases fear of facing the unknown. Emma was unwittingly using the information, not to further her understanding, but to validate her darkest forebodings. Instead of being comforted and reassured by the benign nature of her problem, she was creating a nonexistent problem by conjuring up demons and bogeymen that were threatening to develop a reality of their own.

With each exchange, the gulf of understanding between us seemed to widen. Every explanation I offered somehow became twisted to conform to Emma's conviction that she had a life-threatening illness, and that, for whatever reason, I was being less than candid with her.

Emma's uncanny ability to distort all my attempts at reassurance was disturbing. Despite my concerns for her, I was becoming impatient and frustrated by my inability to communicate with her.

"Have you read anything about the medication that's used to treat mitral valve prolapse? It controls symptoms by blocking the effects of adrenalin."

"No. Will it protect me from having a heart attack?"

"Emma, read my lips. There is no risk of your having a heart attack, so there is no need to protect you from one. The medication is called propranolol. It has been very effective in keeping heart rates from racing, and in mitral valve prolapse patients, it blunts the chest pains and shortness of breath by blocking adrenalin."

"My gynecologist already has me on tranquilizers and sleeping pills to quiet my nervous system."

"Emma, this medication is not a tranquilizer or a sleeping pill. Tranquilizers and sleeping pills act to quiet certain brain functions. Drugs like propranolol are called beta-blockers because they block…"

"Adrenalin. You already told me that. Frankly, they all sound the same to me."

Exasperated, I resorted to what most doctors do. I grabbed my pen, scribbled a prescription for the propranolol, handed it to Emma, and arranged for a return visit in a month to evaluate her response.

Countless mitral valve prolapse patients had come to see me with symptoms similar to Emma's, and over time I was able to calm their fears. Over time, even those with the severe symptoms improved. But never before had I been confronted with a patient like Emma Jorgensen.

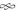

That night, at two o'clock, I was awakened by a call from the emergency room.

The voice on the phone was terse and businesslike. "Got an obese thirty-eight-year-old woman brought in by ambulance complaining of chest pain and shortness of breath. Her physical is normal, and so is everything else, including blood work and electrocardiogram. We've given her a tranquilizer and are ready to send her home, but she says she's your patient and insists on seeing you. That's why I'm calling."

Knowing Emma's medical history, my first thought was to acknowledge the call, and simply have her come to the office the following day, but the situation seemed an ideal opportunity to bridge the chasm that separated us, so I went to see Emma in the ER. By the time I arrived, the tranquilizer had taken hold, and she was no longer having symptoms.

"How are you feeling, Emma?"

"Much better. Thank heavens the ambulance came when it did. I was sure I was a goner."

I did a quick physical, and after scrutinizing the normal electrocardiogram, took Emma's hand.

"I know what you're going to say, Doctor. It's nothing. Just another panic attack in a hysterical patient."

"I wasn't going to say anything of the sort. I'm pleased that everything's okay. Since the starting dose of the beta-blocker doesn't seem to be doing the job, I'm going to increase it."

"Okay, but I don't think it'll do any good."

"It should. I deliberately started you on a low dose. Once we find the right amount, I'm confident that you'll feel a lot better."

Again, Emma's prediction proved better than mine. When I saw her in the office a few days later, she complained of being awakened by shortness of breath for the past several nights.

"Last night, I started to pant so hard that I was sure I was going to pass out. One of these days, it's bound to happen. The next attack could kill me," she said. "When that numb, tingly feeling gets on my hands, and spreads to my face it feels creepy, like I'm being attacked by an invisible alien force from some horror movie."

"The symptoms you're describing are caused by hyperventilation—breathing too rapidly."

"Are you saying that I bring the whole thing on myself? That's not possible. Why do you keep telling me that my problem's in my head?"

Suddenly, an idea came to me. "Emma, I'd like us to do an experiment together. Are you willing?"

"What kind of experiment?"

"I'd like you to breathe as quickly as you can for three minutes. Can you do that?"

"I suppose so."

Emma began warily, and I had to prod her to speed up the breathing. "Make each breath shorter. Pant. Faster. Pretend there's a mad dog chasing after you, and you're running as fast as you can."

After two minutes, Emma said, "I'm beginning to feel sick."

"Keep going," I said, looking at my watch. "You still have another minute to go."

About fifteen seconds later, Emma shrieked, "I have to stop! I'm getting those tingling sensations. I'm going to pass out!"

"Are you having any pain?"

"Not yet."

"Good," I said, putting an arm around her shoulder. "Now take slow, deep breaths. In…out…relax…in…out…"

Emma recovered after a few minutes. "That was awful. Why did you do that to me?"

"I wanted to show you that your breathlessness is not caused by a disease—it's because of the way you breathe when you become anxious. Now I'd like to show you how to breathe so you can avoid having those tingling sensations."

"That was a terrible thing to do, Doctor. You're supposed to make me better, not scare the life out of me."

Persisting with the exercise, I showed Emma that when she breathed, her chest and neck muscles retracted, while her abdomen did not move. I demonstrated how to use her diaphragm, so that her abdomen expanded with each inspiration, and retracted upon expiration. I explained that during a panic attack, she could slow her breathing by pursing her lips while exhaling, as if she were blowing out birthday candles. Although she dutifully followed my directions, Emma seemed to be going through the motions, rather than showing any interest in changing her behavior.

"Put your hands on your abdomen and feel it expand. Breathe all the way in, count one, then exhale," I instructed. "Check the time with your watch. Our goal is for you to take twelve to fourteen breaths per minute. You need to practice this a couple of times a day. It's important."

"I'll try, Doctor."

Two nights later, the emergency room called again. This time the voice on the phone was sharp.

"Your lady is here again. Same symptoms. Same normal physical, EKG, and lab results. When I told her nothing was wrong, she started screaming that she wanted to see her doctor. Are you coming in?"

"All that would do is reinforce her delusion that there's something seriously wrong. Have her call my office in the morning for an appointment."

The following night, Emma was back in the ER. This time the call came from one of the nurses. "Our friend Emergency Emma is back. She says…well, anyway, she's fine. We're sending her home. Just thought you'd want to know."

By the time Emma came to the office at the end of the week, she had been back in the ER two more times, and had made an unscheduled visit to her primary care physician. The situation was spiraling out of control. Emma informed me that her doctor decided to call in reinforcements.

"Dr. Cahill is sending me to a pulmonary specialist. She thinks I might have a lung abnormality that's causing my shortness of breath. The doctor works in her building, so she sent me to his lab for what they call pulmonary function tests, and it turned up a problem. His office told Dr. Cahill that I need a complete evaluation."

"Did anyone tell you what that means?"

"He wants to do a procedure called a bronchoscopy, and a lung biopsy. At this point, I'm so desperate that I'm willing to try anything."

I perused Emma's pulmonary function test results. Her flow rates were normal. That excluded the presence of asthma or obstructive lung disease. No abnormalities were found in the structure or function of her airways. Her lung volumes and ability to exchange oxygen were also normal. The only result in question was a test called the maximum breathing capacity, a study that depends entirely on a patient's cooperation and willingness to breathe as rapidly as possible. In the absence of other abnormal findings, an aberrant result is meaningless. There wasn't a shred of evidence indicating that Emma needed a bronchoscopy.

"Do you know what the procedure entails?" I asked.

"No. Dr. Cahill never explained it to me."

I told Emma that a bronchoscope was a plastic tube that would be inserted down her throat and into her lungs after she had been sedated. The pulmonary doctor would look through the tube for abnormalities, possibly taking biopsies of areas that looked suspicious. Before I could describe the study further, Emma decided that having it was not a good idea.

This was the fourth specialist Emma had seen, and every one of them had done their battery of tests and recommended an invasive procedure. But this was no reason for me to feel superior. I too had been totally ineffective in caring for this woman.

As things grew progressively worse, I suggested lifestyle changes to remedy the situation. I told Emma that she needed to change her diet, eliminating caffeine and all other stimulants, as well as lowering her intake of sweets, because the rapid changes they cause in blood sugar levels are known to trigger the release of adrenalin in susceptible patients. I pressed her to stop taking shots of vodka during the attacks, because alcohol stimulated the heart and could worsen her symptoms. When Emma balked, I offered to make an appointment for her with a dietician.

I also told her to begin an exercise program, beginning with simple walking for twenty to thirty minutes three times a week.

Emma's willingness to share responsibility for her problem by following any of my recommendations was questionable, but when it came to physical activity, she was adamant.

"I'm sorry, Doctor," Emma said, crossing her arms in front of her chest. "Ever since that experience in college, I gave up exercise, and I certainly don't intend to start again now that I'm so sick. Just the thought of it scares me to death."

"I'm not talking about anything strenuous. Why not start with a walk around the block three times a week? Studies have shown that even a little physical activity can reduce the symptoms of mitral valve prolapse."

Emma gave an emphatic shake of her head in tandem with her finger.

When all attempts at lifestyle changes failed, I again resorted to my prescription pad. First, I increased the dose of Emma's propranolol to maximum levels. When that failed to alleviate her symptoms, I changed to a different beta-blocker. When that too failed, I added medications, including a calcium channel blocker.

A vicious cycle was developing. As the frequency and severity of Emma's panic attacks escalated, so too did her preoccupation with her symptoms. They now dominated her life. Emma couldn't bear the thought of having an attack at the library, so she stopped doing volunteer work. It would have been too humiliating.

The next time Emma came to the emergency room, it was for an episode of palpitations.

"My heart rhythm has become chaotic! It's out of control!" she shrieked. When the ER nurse told her that the tracing on the monitor behind her was normal, she replied that the abnormality must have stopped temporarily.

On her following office visit, I ordered a portable electrocardiogram called a Holter monitor. This device makes a tape of the heart rhythm for twenty-four consecutive hours. I asked Emma to write down the specific times when she experienced skipped beats or palpitations, while the EKG was being recorded. Emma indicated three episodes of palpitations. At none of those times was a heart rhythm abnormality present. I showed Emma the results, carefully going over the specific EKG recorded during each instance.

"This should be reassuring," I said. "The test shows that at the time the palpitations occurred, your heart rhythm was normal. Now we can be one hundred percent certain that they are harmless."

Emma shook her head vehemently. "I don't care what that test showed. When those palpitations hit me, it feels like my heart is going to explode. Symptoms that severe can't possibly be harmless."

By now, I had become completely exasperated. "Emma, I know how frightened you are, but frankly, this is too much. Every time I tell you something positive, you question whether or not it's the truth. I've just shown you a conclusive test result, and you say you don't care. I can't be of any use to you if you don't trust what I say. My other patients..."

"I'm not your other patients. I read about my disease and I know what the truth is."

∞

Trust is at the core of the patient-doctor relationship. This includes trust in the doctor's competence, as well as his knowledge and skill, but it also includes trust in *him*—in his commitment, steadfastness, and above all, his word. In Emma's case, communication was the crucial ingredient in her care. But her fear either blocked or distorted all my attempts to alter her morbid obsessions. Whatever the reason, I finally came to realize that I was not going to be of any help to Emma.

My patience had run out. I was tired of trying to take care of this manipulative, controlling woman who knew everything about her disease, and understood nothing.

"Emma, nothing I've done has helped you, and nothing I say seems to register. I think it's time you found yourself another cardiologist. I'm sure Dr. Cahill can suggest someone who will do a better job than I've been able to do."

Tears formed in Emma's eyes. "You mean you want to dump me too? Every doctor I've ever been to can't wait to get me out of the office. No one wants to listen to me. As soon as I start telling them about my illness, they look at their watches and tell me to see their receptionist to schedule some procedure. Even Dr. Cahill has stopped seeing me."

"She has? Since when? Every time you see me, I send her a report. What happened?"

"She told me the same thing you just did. She said she didn't know what else to do for me, or who else to send me to." Emma began sobbing uncontrollably. "I know how difficult I am, and I'm sure you don't like me either, but at least you pay attention to what I'm saying. Please don't abandon me, Doctor! I'll try to be a better patient. Really, I will!"

Emma had more insight than I would have guessed about how difficult a patient she was. And I had to admit that she was right about my not liking her. But I simply could not desert this woman, even though the truth was that I wanted to.

∞

The next morning, the medical director of the emergency room asked to see me.

Striding into my office with an armful of files in hand, Dr. Floyd Field carefully placed them on my desk, staring at me wordlessly. Deep, dark circles, the result of too many sleepless nights on ER duty, accentuated Field's already cadaverous appearance. It was clear that this was not a social visit.

Picking up a sheet of paper from the top of the pile, Field began to rock up and down on his toes while waving it at me.

"You have to do something about Emma Jorgensen," he said. "Do you know how many times she has been to our emergency room in the past two months?"

"I have no idea," I said, "but I'm sure you can tell me."

"Exactly twenty-five times. I lugged her complete ER record over here to make a point. This crazy woman has been a huge pain in the ass. My entire night shift crew is sick of her. I've gotten complaints from the physicians, the nurses, *and* the orderlies who have to drag her fat carcass from the gurney to a bed every time she comes in. Last night, one of the guys told the head nurse that if he had to haul that tub off a gurney one more time, he was going to quit before he got a hernia."

"Floyd, I know better than anyone how difficult Emma is. God knows, I've had my share of problems trying to care for her."

"I'm sorry about that, but I've got my own problems to deal with here. Your patient's ER visits have become a drain on my financial resources as well as my personnel. Every time she comes in, we're obliged to do an electrocardiogram, get a chest x-ray, and a battery of blood tests even though they are a waste of time and money. It's standard procedure to protect ERs from malpractice suits. One time, some fancy-pants intern got the bright idea that your patient might have an aortic tear, so he took it on himself to order an MRI."

"I understand your problem, and I'll do my best to get Emma to…"

"Your best just isn't good enough. The hospital has cut my budget to the bone, and we need every penny to take care of the people who really need help."

∞

One week later, Emma was in a supermarket when a major incident occurred. As she stood in line at the checkout counter, her heart began to speed up and she became short of breath. The line was moving slowly, and the longer she stood there, the worse her symptoms became.

"Did you try taking those deep breaths we practiced in the office?" I asked.

"No, the thought never occurred to me. I was too scared. My face and hands were tingling, and I felt weak all over, like I was going to faint right in front of all those people, so I left the shopping cart and pushed through the line while everyone stared at me. I managed to reach the street, and collapsed on a nearby bench.

"People going in and out of the market were sneaking looks at me, but no one offered to help. It was so humiliating. After a few minutes I decided to see if I could get home.

"I really don't know how, but I did it. My house is only two blocks from the store, but it took me more than an hour. I'm sure the people who saw me thought I was a crazy drunk, inching along, and clinging to the walls of buildings. The hardest part was getting across the street. I was afraid I was going to fall down and get hit by a car."

"What did you do when you got home?"

"What I always do. Took a fistful of tranquilizers, and went to bed."

"A fistful of tranquilizers? That's dangerous, Emma! Why didn't you call 911?"

"Because the people in the emergency room can't stand me. I didn't know how they'd react if I showed up during the day. Thank heaven, Gladys, my next-door neighbor, saw me trying to get in my front door. She came over to make sure I was okay, and brought along some nice hot cocoa. When I told her my story, Gladys was horrified because she knows I have a heart condition. She said when I get an attack like that, I should *always* call 911. 'Too bad about those terrible ER people,' she said. Gladys is so sweet. She volunteered to drive me here today."

I left Emma's exam room and was making my way past the reception area, when I was accosted by a fleshy woman in a faded housedress, with thin gray hair pulled back in a bun, and a flat nose displaying a large mole on the left side. Looking me over, she said in an East European accent, "Pardon me, Doctor, my name is Gladys Lovatna. I'm Emma's next-door neighbor."

Before I could respond, she continued. "I have to talk to you. That poor girl has no one but me. Both her parents are gone. Her sister lives in Australia, and they haven't spoken in years. What she's been going through is criminal, and none of those other doctors did a thing for her. If you don't find a way to make that girl better soon, Doctor, it's going to be too late. She's getting worse all the time. When Emma came back from the supermarket, she looked like a ghost. I don't know how she made it home. You'll help her won't you, Doctor?"

"I'll do everything I can," I said, searching for a pleasant way to end this meeting. "It's nice to have met you, Gladys."

Ignoring my attempt to leave, she continued, "I told Emma that whenever she gets one of those terrible attacks, she shouldn't even think twice about going to the ER. I'm sure you agree, don't you, Doctor?"

I was not about to engage this woman with a detailed explanation of Emma's medical condition. Smiling vaguely, I thanked her for her concern, and fled.

∞

After the supermarket episode, Emma's life changed drastically. Afraid to leave the house, she became immobilized, spending endless days shuffling from room to room, wearing the same terrycloth robe, taking long baths to soothe herself, and weeping in despair of the coming darkness, when the inevitable symptoms would assail her. Afraid to sleep for fear of being awakened by another attack, Emma spent entire nights sitting in the kitchen, devouring quarts of Ben and Jerry's ice cream and boxes of Oreo cookies.

The only time she left her home was when Gladys came over, helped her into the car, and drove her to the office.

"My weight is out of control," Emma admitted during one such visit, after the scale showed a gain of twenty pounds in two months, "but food is the only thing that keeps me from losing my sanity."

I made another change in Emma's beta-blocker medication, and increased the dose of her calcium blocker drug, but I was not expecting any breakthroughs. The truth was that Emma was testing me in ways no patient had ever done before, and I was failing her. I suggested that Emma see a hypnotherapist. When she again insisted that the trouble was her heart and not her head, I became adamant, insisting that Emma at least see the therapist for a consultation. Finally nodding in reluctant agreement, Emma took my note with the doctor's name and telephone number, silently tucked it into her purse, and left the office.

After being housebound for more than a month, there was a sudden drop-off in the frequency of Emma's emergency room visits. Had a miracle happened? Had those changes in Emma's beta-blocker and calcium blocker medications somehow managed to control her symptoms at long last? Desperation had driven me into a fantasyland of my own.

Reality reasserted itself when Emma arrived for her next appointment.

"Doctor, I've come to say good-bye. This will be the last time I see you."

"Why is that, Emma?"

"I am going to die."

In contrast to her usual agitated, frantic manner of speech, Emma made her declaration in a flat, matter-of-fact tone. At first, I thought she was depressed, or drugged out by tranquilizers. But when her eyes met mine, they were steady and unwavering for the first time.

"What are you saying, Emma? You're not thinking about..."

"No, Doctor. I'm not planning to commit suicide. But I am certain that my time has come."

Reflexively, I grabbed the box of tissues on my desk, anticipating the inevitable tears, but Emma remained calm and composed. Gone were the wild gesticulations, the staccato flashings of her flabby arms waving about to convey the enormity of what was befalling her. Emma displayed no emotion whatsoever.

This was not the first time a patient had told me that death was imminent. Usually, it occurred when the final stage of their disease had been reached. Occasionally, a patient seemed to intuit impending death despite every indication of a good prognosis. And despite the corroborative medical data of a benign angiogram, electrocardiogram, scan, and blood tests, the patient's prediction frequently proved accurate. I had long ago learned to take these pronouncements seriously.

While Emma's belief that she would soon die was compelling, from a medical standpoint, there seemed no reason for concern. Every patient who made this ominous prediction previously had a serious illness.

I reached out and took hold of Emma's hands.

"I know how you've been suffering..."

"No, Doctor, you don't. No one will ever know," she said evenly.

"That may be true, but please believe me. You are *not* going to die."

Emma's hands hung heavily in mine. She seemed far away.

"I'm sorry I've been such a burden to you and your staff, Doctor. The people in the emergency room did their best, even though they thought I was a pathetic pig."

"Emma, the emergency room staff…"

"It's okay, Doctor. All of you tried, but everyone either pities me or thinks I should be committed to a fat farm or an insane asylum. I never told you this, but I heard one of the nurses say 'oink, oink' while they were wheeling me down the hall on one of my ER visits. They even have a nickname for me: 'Emergency Emma.'"

"That's unforgivable! Why didn't you tell me?"

"There's no need to bother with that now. The people in the emergency room will be relieved not to have to drag two-ton Emma from the gurney to a bed, or struggle trying to get a blood pressure cuff around my big, fat arms. That ugly scenario is over. I know you'd never admit it, Doctor, but you'll be relieved too."

"That's not true, Emma."

A knowing smile broke briefly over Emma's face before it returned to its emotionless mask. "You've meant well, Doctor. Really, there's no need for you to feel guilty about anything."

"Emma, you've had these episodes countless times. Why would you think the next one is going to kill you?"

"Because my luck has run out. And please, no more speeches about how benign my condition is, or if I'd only do this or that, everything will be fine." Emma stood up and put out her hand to shake mine. "Good-bye," she said.

This was no act by Emma, the drama queen. But I knew her medical condition was benign, and that it posed no threat. Why, then, did I need to reassure myself? Did I sense something in Emma that gave credence to her dire prediction? Was my impotence and abysmal failure to care for this desperate, lonely woman talking? These questions plagued me throughout the night.

The following day, I called Emma's house. When she did not answer, I left a message. When she did not return the call, I made several more attempts. All were futile.

Weeks passed and still Emma did not call, make office appointments, or visit the emergency room. I thought about calling 911, but felt that it would probably result in another false alarm. Perhaps Gladys had prevailed on her neighbor to move in with her. Perhaps Emma went to see another doctor. Over the next several months, I called occasionally, but never received a reply.

∞

Eight months later, I was finishing some paperwork prior to seeing office patients, when my receptionist called on the intercom. "Dr. H., when you have a minute, would you please come over? Someone is here to see you."

"One of the new patients?"

"No, an old patient."

I did not recognize the handsome woman with auburn hair, dressed in a tan suit and matching shoes standing at the reception desk. Her knowing eyes sparkled as she approached me.

"Do I have to introduce myself, Doctor?" she said smiling.

Only when I heard her voice did I realize who it was. "Emma? Is it really you? I can't believe my eyes," I said, giving her a big hug.

"At times, it's hard for me to believe too."

"I'm relieved to see that your prediction was wrong after all," I said, once we were in my office.

"Prediction? About what?"

"You were certain that you were going to die."

"Oh yes. Do you want to know what happened?"

"I sure would. I was quite concerned, when you didn't return my calls."

"The night after my last office visit, I had another bout of palpitations, followed by shortness of breath. But the chest pain that came after that was different from the others. It was far more intense and frightening. As usual, I went straight to bed, put a pillow over my chest, and got into a fetal position, but that only made my breathing worse.

"So I got up and did what I always do. I went into the kitchen, and emptied the refrigerator. Gorging usually made me feel better, but not that night. I remembered the vodka in the freezer, and took a few nips hoping it would do the trick. When that didn't work, I went to the bathroom, got out the tranquilizers and sleeping pills, put a bunch in my hand, and gulped them down."

"My god! What were they?"

"I don't know. Xanax, Valium, whatever I could find. Anything that might give me some relief. But they didn't work either."

"Why didn't you call, or come to the emergency room?"

"I thought about that of course, but the last time I was there, the nurses paged Dr. Field, the head ER doctor. He came over and started unloading on me. He scolded me right in front of the entire staff for wasting their time and resources, and practically ordered me never to come back. I was mortified. Believe me, I really wanted to call 911 and go to the ER that night, but I couldn't bear the thought of facing those people again."

"I can't believe Dr. Field would say something like that to you. Don't you think you might be exaggerating a little?"

"I have no reason to exaggerate anything. The staff there was sick and tired of me and my false alarms, and you were too, Doctor. I always knew you thought I was a pain in the neck."

"It's true that you were a pain, but I did care about you, Emma. I wanted to help, but everything I tried failed."

"It's okay, Doctor. I don't blame you. Every physician I saw reacted the same way. All of you thought I was a hopeless hypochondriac."

"I became frustrated because I was trying to help you, and couldn't. Please go on with your story."

"By now, I was exhausted and I began to panic. I kept telling myself to breathe more slowly, and I tried to take deep inhalations, pursing my lips the way you showed me, but I couldn't get enough air."

"What did you do then?"

"I decided to take a hot bath. Sometimes that relaxes me. I took another shot of vodka, and slid in. The water was scalding, but it soothed me, and I began to relax. The air in the room became thick and steamy, like a Turkish bath. Everything became gray and fuzzy, like a sort of twilight zone. I must have fallen asleep, but after a while, I felt the palpitations again, and woke up. Each heartbeat felt like a sledgehammer pounding through the fog. Then the shortness of breath returned, but it was different from anything I'd ever experienced before.

"This time, no matter how hard I tried, it seemed like I couldn't get any air. Prior to this, I'd been having recurring nightmares that I was going to suffocate to death, and now it was happening. Everything became dense and murky. I sensed a bubbling sensation in my lungs. The thought came to me that maybe I was underwater, and was drowning. I tried to lift myself up, but between my breathlessness, the pounding in my chest, and my bulk, I couldn't move. It was hopeless. I was going to die. Then, something incredible happened.

"I felt like I was being lifted out of my body, and I realized that it was really happening. This was really it. I was dying. The incredible part was that it seemed perfectly okay. When that realization struck me, everything became calm. I felt weightless, as if the burdens I had been lugging around for so long had vanished. Not just the weight of my body, but the weight of my life."

"Were you afraid?"

"Not at all. It was quite matter-of-fact, and strangely comforting. I had spent my life consumed by a fear of death, and when the moment finally arrived, I was at peace."

"So you accepted the inevitable?"

"I didn't just accept it, I welcomed it! I was suspended in this exquisite state, and all I wanted was to continue the voyage. Everything was fluid, as though I had dissolved in the water. No form. No fear. No *me*. I was free. It was exhilarating."

"What about your symptoms?"

"They were still present in a vague sort of way, but they no longer concerned me. Then, I heard a voice. I'm not a religious person, Doctor, but it was as clear as your voice is now. It said, 'Your life is a gift. Use it wisely.' Then the fog began to clear, and I realized that my head was no longer under the water. I was alive, and breathing air."

"How did you feel?"

"It was deeply depressing. Sort of like I had been free, and now I was back in the dreary dungeon of my life. That's when I realized how my obsession with death had prevented me from being truly alive. I had no friends. I had never been loved and had never really loved anyone, including my sister and ex-husband. And, I had never done anything worthwhile. All my energy was spent walling myself off from the world.

"I had to die to appreciate life. Now that I've discovered that death is nothing to be feared, I want to open to life as fully as possible."

Emma's once quivery voice now conveyed a depth and richness that matched the serenity in her eyes. Instead of sagging in the chair, she sat comfortably, displaying none of her former agitation. Her body remained upright and quiet while her hands rested in her lap. When Emma smiled, her face lit up with a gentle sweetness.

"You look fantastic, Emma," I said. "How did you manage to take off all that weight? You must have lost a hundred pounds."

"One hundred and twenty-two to be exact. Once I started sleeping at night, instead of eating the refrigerator, the weight just seemed to melt away. Of course, eliminating the Ben and Jerry's and the Oreo cookies helped too." A smile filled Emma's eyes. "I also began walking. You were right about exercise. I'd forgotten how good it feels."

"Emma, you are a very courageous woman."

Emma put her hands together and looked at me thoughtfully. "I don't want to make it sound as if everything happened overnight. I eased my way into the world, literally a step at a time. The first day I left the house, I made it to the driveway, stopped, took a couple of deep breaths, and went back. After a few days, I made it to the corner of my block. Then, it was two blocks. It took two weeks before the big breakthrough: going to the market. But I did it."

"Do you still have symptoms?"

"Occasionally, but my relationship with them has changed. Before, when they appeared, I'd be overcome by fear. Now when they occur, I notice them, and that's all. That's been another interesting discovery.

When I let my symptoms be, they let me be. I go about my business, and they pass."

"Not even a little fear?"

"At times, but I've explored my fear and I've explored myself. I've always wanted to help people. That's why I liked working in the library. But now, I think I can use my experience to help your patients."

"Really? What do you have in mind?"

"Most of your patients are fear-ridden, and although they usually have good reasons to be, my guess is that most of them have no one to talk to about it."

Emma looked at me with a mischievous grin. "Don't get me wrong, Doctor. You and your staff are well meaning, but you're busy people. The few minutes you give your patients is helpful, but some of them need more. They're isolated and alone, and no one knows better than I that the more helpless and frightened people feel, the more frantic their minds become. I'm not suggesting that I become their priest or therapist or anything like that, but I can be a good listener, and I can be there for them. Please give it some thought."

Could this open, engaging woman once have been my panic-ridden patient? Perhaps Emma's experience with death had given her insights that could be helpful to some of my patients. After all, she had already provided me with several insights. Too often, I tried to talk my patients out of their fears instead of first acknowledging their presence. Maybe I have been too busy trying to find a solution, and don't always take the time to really *be* with them.

One of my patients in the coronary care unit had a problem that was baffling me, and I sensed that a visit from Emma might be helpful. Joan was a fifty-eight-year-old woman who had been admitted to the unit with a heart attack. The attack was minor, but when I told her the good news, she showed no emotion and simply looked away. Unexpected complications soon set in. Every few hours, a burst of rapid, irregular heartbeats occurred, accompanied by skyrocketing blood pressures. At first, the heart rhythm disturbances responded to medication, but then they recurred and began to increase. Tests were unable to provide a reason for these episodes.

Throughout her illness, Joan refused to make eye contact, remaining mute whenever I attempted to discuss her situation. I thought it unlikely that she would want to meet with anyone, but when I introduced her to Emma, the two women somehow connected and Joan immediately agreed to a visit.

Three days later, I asked Emma to see me. For twenty-four hours, my patient had not had an episode of rapid heart rate, rhythm irregularity, or blood pressure elevation. While assuming no connection, I was curious about what had taken place during Emma's visits.

"The first thing Joan told me was that she wasn't going to make it out of the hospital. When I asked why, she told me about her mother's heart attack. It seems that when Joan's mother first began to have the chest pains, Joan tried to reassure her that they were harmless by repeating the common belief that women didn't get heart attacks. Several hours later, her mother was dead. Ever since then, Joan's been certain that she too would have a heart attack and die, just like her mother."

"What did you say to convince her otherwise?"

"I didn't say anything. I just listened. Joan had never told her story to anyone, and as soon as she began to unburden herself, the tears poured out. At first, I was concerned that she would get one of those irregular heartbeat episodes, but it seemed that she was freeing herself from the guilt that had kept her in its grasp for so many years."

Emma's ability to listen openheartedly to patients provided a welcome opportunity for them to unburden themselves. Without judging or questioning the validity of their feelings, Emma gently suggested that, like her, they could choose to view their illness as an opportunity to make peace with themselves, and to heal the past. She laughed with them, cried with them, and most importantly, became a friend, an ally, and an invaluable source of comfort and support.

In Emma's words, "Dying was the greatest thing that almost happened to me."

The Priest

"I am certain of nothing...."
—W. B. Yeats

"Sorry to bother you," Dr. Kennedy said over the phone, "but last night, my priest had some discomfort in one of his arms. It seemed to come and go, but it kept him up most of the night. He came in to see me this morning, and while I didn't find anything specific, I'd appreciate it if you would come over and take a quick look before I send him on his way."

Mike Kennedy was an internist, and president of the hospital medical staff. Over the years, we had worked closely on a number of hospital and medical school matters. In the eight years since I had joined the medical center, this was the first time Mike Kennedy had ever asked me to see an office patient. Slipping into a lab coat, I quickly headed to his office in the adjoining building of the hospital complex.

When I arrived, Mike nodded toward the far side of the office, where a man wearing a collarless white shirt, pressed black slacks, and black wing-tip shoes sat on a leather sofa with his arms wound tightly across his chest. "I'd like you to meet my priest, Father John More."

"Nice to meet you, Father," I said.

"Likewise, Doctor," he replied pleasantly.

Mike continued, "I've been John's doctor for years, and except for high blood pressure, he's always been in good health. Anyway, as I told you on the phone, he woke up in the middle of the night with a strange discomfort in his arm. I'm sure he's okay, but something…"

"But nothing," Father More said, grinning broadly. "It was most kind of you to come over, Doctor, but I'm afraid your visit is quite unnecessary. Michael should not have bothered you."

Father More rose, while continuing to keep both arms wrapped around his tall, angular frame. The priest's tight smile seemed to be as permanently fixed to the landscape of his craggy face as its hollow cheekbones, thin lips, and angular nose. Deep, dark trenches were carved into his forehead.

Reaching out to shake his hand, I said, "You're probably right, Father, but since I'm already here, maybe I could ask you a few questions, and briefly examine you."

"Michael has already examined me, and as you can see, I've dressed," he said with practiced politeness. While looking at me with pale, piercing eyes, he put on a black suit jacket.

"It'll only take a minute," I said.

"Please don't trouble yourself any further, Doctor," he replied, while impatiently brushing off two errant hairs that had fallen on the jacket from his meticulously groomed white mane. "Thank you again, but I'm already late for an important church meeting. Good-bye."

As he moved toward the door, Father More reached back and belatedly extended his hand to meet mine. In that moment, everything changed.

It was a warm spring day, and sunlight streamed in through an open window. Yet my hand felt as though it was grasping icy tentacles. Father More's palm was unaccountably wet. Looking closely at his face, I saw that it had become mottled, and was as white and pasty as his shirt. Beads of perspiration were forming on his brow. Alarm bells began ringing in my head.

"I'd better sit down for a minute," Father More said, moving back toward the couch. "I feel a little weak. That pain in my arm is back. Damn thing kept me up most of the night."

"Which arm is bothering you?" I asked.

"The left one. Why does that matter?"

"Sometimes pain in the left arm can be coming from the heart. It's known as referred pain. Did you have any discomfort in your chest last night, Father?"

"No. If there had been, I certainly would have told Michael."

"Any shortness of breath?"

"A little. Mostly, I feel cold, and sweaty. It's probably some kind of virus."

Determined to press on, I took a stethoscope out of my lab coat pocket. This man was almost certainly in the midst of a serious heart attack. "Father, I really need to examine your chest."

"Is this really necessary, Michael?" Father More said, turning to Dr. Kennedy. "I just feel weak. A little rest and I'm sure everything will be fine."

But Mike had begun to look apprehensive. "I did find that John's blood pressure was lower than normal. Usually, it runs about 145 over 95. Today, it was only 115 over 80." Mike turned to his patient. "John, please..."

"All right, but please make it quick. As I said, I have important work to do at church today," Father More said, while removing his jacket and unbuttoning his shirt. His breathing was becoming labored, and sweat was now pouring off his brow.

As soon as I placed the stethoscope over Father More's heart, my concern skyrocketed. It was racing at 140 beats per minute—almost twice normal. In addition, an abnormal heart sound called a gallop, unmistakable evidence of a failing heart, was clearly audible.

Moving the stethoscope to Father More's back, I listened to his lungs. My ears were filled with gurgling noises called rales. That meant fluid was accumulating in Father More's lungs—a dangerous sign that his breathing difficulty was being caused by heart failure. Father More's chest felt cold and clammy, and his pulse was weak and thready. Sweat now exploded over his entire body. When I rolled up Father More's sleeve to take his blood pressure, he made no attempt to resist. The pressure was down to 90 over 60. Father More's circulatory system was collapsing before my eyes.

"My arm feels like it's in a vise," he said miserably, as I put the stethoscope back in my lab coat.

"I'm sorry to have to tell you this, Father, but it's pretty clear that you're having a heart attack. We need to get a confirmatory electrocardiogram, and admit you to the coronary care unit right away. The sooner we can begin…"

"I can't be having a heart attack. It's just a bad case of the flu." Holding his left arm, Father More turned to Dr. Kennedy.

While the priest's eyes cried out in fear, his mind could not accept the enormity of what was happening to him. It was as if he had barricaded himself inside a house that was in flames. I had to break in before the blaze consumed him.

Father More needed to be on a monitor with an intravenous line so he could be given medication to combat the rapidly accumulating pulmonary fluid. As Father More's lungs became more flooded, critically needed oxygen would soon be prevented from reaching his bloodstream. A vicious cycle of increased cardiac damage and heart failure might result. I too turned to Dr. Kennedy for support.

"Mike, Father More has a loud gallop, and wet rales halfway up both lungs. His pressure is down. This is a major coronary until proven otherwise. We need to move quickly."

"None of those abnormalities were present on my physical just a half hour ago," Mike said. "The attack must have begun in the last few minutes." Putting a hand on Father More's shoulder, he said, "We can confirm the diagnosis in just a few minutes, John, but you really must have the electrocardiogram. It's essential."

"Please go along with us at least that far, Father," I said.

"That far, and that far only."

∞

Although the most common symptom of a heart attack is severe, crushing pain in the center of the chest, the discomfort may occur in the left or both shoulders, arms, or wrists, as well as the upper abdomen, the lower jaw, and even in the center of the back. Weakness, sweating, nausea, and a sense of impending doom often accompany the attack. Although the most common presenting complaint is pain, it is not always present. In patients with diabetes, or in the elderly, as many as 50 percent of heart attacks may be painless.

In most cases, a heart attack occurs when an atherosclerotic, cholesterol-filled plaque in one of the coronary arteries ruptures. A clot (also called a thrombus, hence the term coronary thrombosis) then forms on the exposed plaque area, abruptly occluding the blood vessel. In the initial stages, the clot may be incomplete, and patients experience transient, recurring pains before the occlusion becomes permanent. That was what had happened to Father More.

Once a coronary artery occlusion occurs, the patient's prognosis depends on the extent of the cardiac area in jeopardy. When this area is substantial, the heart becomes incapable of pumping sufficient amounts of blood to the body. If the cardiac output decreases significantly, the patient's blood pressure drops, reducing blood supply to the vital bodily organs and impairing their ability to function—a condition called shock.

Today, we would open the blocked artery with an angioplasty balloon or clot buster medication. But at that time, we did not have the ability to open the blocked artery, making it impossible to rescue the jeopardized area of Father More's heart. Our only option was to treat the effects of the failing heart, and hope that either the clot would dissolve on its own, or that the damage would be small enough to allow him to survive. Then, after his heart healed, the odds were that it would function well enough to allow him to live a normal life. In most heart attack victims, that was what occurred. But on Father More's physical examination, all the evidence indicated that his heart attack was massive.

∞

Moving to the phone, I said to Mike, "I'll call ahead to the EKG lab. Let's get a gurney so we can wheel Father More..."

"You're not going to wheel me through the hall like a pathetic invalid," Father More said in a weakened voice.

Within minutes, Father More was in the heart station. One glance at the electrocardiogram confirmed my worst fears.

∞

In a patient with a major heart attack, electrocardiogram abnormalities are usually unmistakable. Father More's electrocardiogram showed astronomical elevations of the ST segment and pathologic Q waves. These abnormalities indicated that the area of the heart under attack was both widespread and had already penetrated deep into the affected muscle layers.

I focused on what we could do. Step one was to relieve the flooded lungs caused by heart failure. Intravenous morphine and diuretic medications were usually effective. It was also crucial to keep a vigilant eye on Father More's heart rhythm. In the first hours of a heart attack, the biggest threat to a patient's life is a catastrophic breakdown of the heartbeat called ventricular fibrillation, more commonly called a cardiac arrest. The majority of patients who die before they reach the hospital succumb because of a cardiac arrest.

Coronary care units were created to detect ominous harbingers of arrest in heart attack victims called premature ventricular beats. When these beats are quickly spotted on a monitor and treated with an intravenous medication called lidocaine, the heart rhythm can usually be normalized before the arrest occurs.

∞

"Father," I said, "I'm afraid the EKG has confirmed that you're having a serious heart attack. We need to get you to the coronary care unit immediately. The sooner we begin treating you, the better."

Holding his arm, his breathing increasingly labored, Father More silently acquiesced. I hastily assembled a transport team of two nurses and an orderly. We attached our new patient to a portable cardiac monitor, and started an intravenous through which we gave him a dose of morphine to ease his pain, and a diuretic drug to combat the accumulating pulmonary fluid.

As we began wheeling him to the unit, an outbreak of premature ventricular beats suddenly appeared on the monitor. Unless treated immediately, they could degenerate into a cardiac arrest.

"He's having runs of premature beats!" I said. "Get one hundred milligrams of lidocaine into the IV line."

But within seconds, the cardiac rhythm became completely chaotic. It was ventricular fibrillation—a cardiac arrest. The priest's heart stopped contracting, and he lost consciousness.

"Call a code!" I shouted, as I began cardiopulmonary resuscitation, tearing off Father More's shirt and rhythmically pounding on his breastbone to try to keep blood circulating to his body.

Within minutes, the arrest team arrived. "Charge the defibrillator," I ordered, stepping away from my patient as the nurses placed the electrode paddles on Father More's chest.

"It's charged," someone behind me said.

"Clear," I said, turning toward the monitor as the electrical discharge jolted Father More's inert body. A slow, halting rhythm began to bleep across the screen. Riveted to each beat, I tried to will the rhythm back to normal. Father More's heart would not contract normally unless the beat quickened. A dose of adrenalin might speed the rate, but that risked throwing it back into fibrillation. Inserting a temporary pacemaker would take too much time. While my mind frantically searched for other alternatives, I stared at the monitor. The beat began to quicken.

"Check the blood pressure," I said, eyes still glued to the monitor.

"I can barely get it. Sixty over zero."

He's breathing spontaneously," someone said. Looking down, I saw that my patient was breathing on his own. We're out of the woods, I said to myself, but when I turned back to the monitor, bursts of irregular heartbeats were again present. Another cardiac arrest was imminent.

"One-hundred-milligram push of intravenous lidocaine, now. Do it!" I shouted.

"In," came the reply. With one set of eyes, the team stared at the monitor screen. Had the medication been given in time? Would it restrain the irregular beats before they again raged out of control? Slowly, they began to disappear.

"What's the pressure now?" I asked.

"Better. Up to 80 over 60."

"Okay, let's get him to the unit. Where's Norman?"

"Right here."

Dr. Norman Katz was one of our best cardiology trainees. Already certified in internal medicine at Montefiore Medical Center in New York City, he had come to the Philadelphia Heart Institute to get his boards in cardiology. Norman was one of my favorites. While he had the style, strut, and swagger of a New Yorker, Norman was a superb doctor.

"Norman, I'm going to stay with Father More. You get over to the unit and set up for him, okay?"

"You got it."

By the time Father More's monitors, blood pressure apparatus, and intravenous were reattached in the coronary care unit, he had begun to regain consciousness. In a groggy voice, he asked what happened.

"You've had a cardiac arrest, Father, but you're stable now. We have you in the coronary care unit, and the nurses here are the best. They'll take good care of you."

"Strange," Father More said. "I felt like I was looking down at all of you while you were working on me. There were beautiful sounds...like some sort of lovely music. I don't know how to describe it...so quiet...so...peaceful..." Slowly he trailed off.

"You've been through a lot, Father. It would be good to rest now."

I paid no attention to these strange mumblings. At that moment, Father More's tenuous medical condition consumed me. My sole concern was making certain that his vital signs remained stable. While the nurses administered additional morphine and Lasix medications to treat the persistent fluid in Father More's lungs, I focused on his heart rhythm and blood pressure monitors.

∞

Dr. Kennedy was pacing at the nurses' station when I came out of Father More's room. "How's John doing? Is he going to be all right?"

"It's too early to tell. He's had a massive coronary, and I have a feeling we're going to have our hands full."

"Well, I'll leave him in your care."

After Kennedy left, I sat down beside Carole Waters, the unit head nurse, to write an admission note and treatment orders. Carole was a short, heavyset woman in her late thirties. She used little makeup, and cared nothing about physical appearances, but her deep brown eyes radiated a loving-kindness that lit up her cherubic face. Carole was a healer.

The nurses who worked for this woman revered her, while the interns, residents, and cardiology trainees somewhat grudgingly admired her daunting clinical skills. Her astute observations and quiet suggestions to the unit doctors were invaluable. Carole always seemed to know.

Carole and I had a long-established professional bond and a mutual commitment to caring for our patients. Both of us were dedicated to instilling the unique responsibilities of our calling into the cadres of nurses, doctors, and students who rotated through the coronary care unit.

Recently, strange reading material had begun to appear on Carole's desk: books about metaphysical healing, Chinese chi massage, and Native American shamanism. When I asked Carole about her new interests, she refused to discuss them, telling me with an amused look that I wasn't ready.

As I began scribbling a note on the chart, Carole said, "I have bad vibes about Father More. His blood pressure and cardiac output are low, and I think he's in borderline shock. What do you think about using the intra-aortic balloon?"

∞

An intra-aortic balloon counterpulsation pump is a machine that temporarily assists the heart. The balloon on the front end of a long plastic catheter tube is threaded through the groin and into the main artery, the aorta.

The counterpulsation is a rhythmic expanding and deflating of the balloon in sync with the heart contractions. This helps a damaged heart to pump more blood, while at the same time allowing it to do less work. As the heart mends itself sufficiently, its performance improves, and the patient can gradually be weaned from the pump.

But this lifesaving machine was also a time bomb. After about a week, the device usually begins to cause devastating side effects, such as destroying the patient's red blood cells or causing lethal bacterial infections. Either development leaves no alternative but to remove it, even if a patient's heart has not recovered. Even if the patient's continued survival depends on it. Once inserted, the counterpulsation balloon would compel us to begin a grim race with time.

∞

"Don't you think that's jumping the gun a bit?" I said. "I'm not sure we need to go there. Not yet anyway. Let's see what happens after his lungs clear and his rhythm stabilizes."

"Okay, but I have a feeling…"

"I hear you, Carole, but with any luck, he'll settle down."

"Well, Father More should be able to call on more than luck. After all, he has a direct line to the Higher Power."

By late afternoon, Father More had begun to stabilize. His heart rhythm remained regular. His blood pressure stayed low, but was adequate. Having slept more than three hours, Father More was now fully awake.

"How are you feeling, Father?" I asked.

"Like I've been hit by a truck. What happened to me?"

"You've had a heart attack, Father. At the moment, your condition is stable, but we're going to have to keep a close eye on things."

"How long do I have to stay here? This is a terribly busy time for me at the church. I have urgent business to attend to."

"It's too early to say, Father. But I promise we won't keep you a minute longer than necessary."

"Pardon me for saying so, but that's a typical doctor answer. Why do you physicians have to be so evasive? If I was that fuzzy-minded with my parishioners…" Trailing off, Father More closed his eyes.

"Father, I wish I could be less vague, but at this point, it's too soon to know," I said, too loudly in my frustration.

∞

Much as I hated to admit it, Father More was right. Doctors are vague and evasive far too often—and far too often, we are embarrassed and in denial about how little we really know. I had no idea what Father More's outcome would be, and the uncertainty was deeply disturbing. I was responsible for the life of this sick man, and did not know if I could save him.

∞

Early that evening, I stopped by the coronary care unit to check on my patients before leaving the hospital. Father More was sitting up in bed, looking much improved. His lungs sounded clear, free of edema fluid, and the heart gallop, though still audible, had softened. His blood pressure remained stable at 90 over 60, with only a few scattered extra beats detected on the EKG monitor. After I completed his exam, Father More pressed me again about discharging him from the hospital.

"You don't fully understand the importance of my work, and how much my parishioners depend on me. They need my guidance," he said, "and when necessary, a swift kick in the rear. But I'm always there for them. Michael knows."

"Father, I know how important you are to a lot of people, but before you can help them, you need to get well. You have my word that we'll get you back to your church as quickly as possible. You've been through a lot, and I'm sure it's been a terrible shock, but right now, the best thing you can do is to get a good night's rest. I'll call Dr. Kennedy and let him know how pleased we are with your progress. He's been concerned about you."

"Good. And while you're at it, please tell Michael I want to see him right away."

As I picked up a phone at the nurses' station, two concerns preoccupied me. Father More had stabilized after his cardiac arrest, and on the surface, everything seemed to be going remarkably well, but the blood tests confirmed that a substantial amount of damage had occurred. After a heart attack, cardiac proteins referred to as CPK and SGOT are released into the blood from the damaged muscle. The amounts released provide a reasonably reliable estimate of the damage. Father More's CPK and SGOT blood levels were both sky high.

Added to that was the second concern: Father More's refusal to accept the seriousness of his illness. The priest's obsession with church matters seemed to have made him incapable of acknowledging what had happened. Rather than call, I decided to stop by Mike Kennedy's office to discuss the situation.

I filled Mike in on the medical details and told him about my concerns.

"I'm sure that once I see John, I'll be able to convince him to accept the situation," he said. "I know dealing with John can be tough. I'm on the church board, and believe me, he gets pretty intense at some of those meetings.

"Father's an old-fashioned priest, and an old-fashioned disciplinarian, but I'll tell you one thing. Even though I think John can overdo the hell-fire and damnation stuff, I have enormous respect for the sincerity of his convictions. The man has devoted his life to Christ and his parish.

"Right now, John's terrified. The orderliness of his life has been destroyed. But he'll calm down after I talk with him. I've known him a long time, and we're good friends. I'd like to I tell you a story about John, so you can understand him a little better. Okay?"

"Sure."

"Please keep this to yourself. The only reason I know about this is because both of us strayed a bit beyond our usual allotment of fine Irish whisky one night, after a particularly tense board meeting. Father got a little loose and unburdened himself.

"John had an awful childhood. He was a shy, sensitive boy who preferred reading to sports or being in the rough and tumble of the streets. But his father was a tyrannical Irish cop who took sadistic pleasure from regularly thrashing the hell out of his son.

"When he was six years old, John tried to run away from home after a particularly severe beating. He returned that same night, cold and hungry, having gotten as far as a block away. His father gave him another beating, and locked him in his room. For three days, the boy was given one glass of water, and no food.

"Each morning before leaving for work, his father would unlock John's door. He'd enter the room dressed in his police uniform with a belt in his hand, force John to strip, and beat him senseless. When he returned in the evening, the man would beat his son again, and then give him the glass of water. After each whipping, the boy was forced to thank his father for caring enough to punish him for his own good. Only then could John drink his glass of water.

"On the second day, John was told he could no longer scream during the beatings. Instead, he was to say thank you after each blow. By the end of the third day, he had collapsed into a semiconscious stupor."

"What a nightmarish thing for a child to endure. It's amazing he survived. He must have hated that sadistic bastard."

"The story doesn't end there. A few months later, John's father began to complain about pains in his arms. When his wife suggested that he see a doctor, her advice was scorned. But the boy sensed that something was seriously wrong with his father."

"Two days later, on a bitter wintry day, John's father walked out the front door of the house, holding his arm. He never returned."

"Died of a heart attack, I'll bet."

"He collapsed a couple of hours later, during a poker game with his buddies at the station. They tried to resuscitate him, but…"

"How did John react to his father's death?"

"He said it was the defining moment of his life. John made the decision to devote his life to Christ at his father's funeral."

"Did he believe God struck down his father?"

"John refused to talk about that."

∞

The following morning, Norman greeted me with a smile.

"Father More's a lot better. Blood pressure's up, heart rhythm's stable, no gallop, and no fluid in his lungs. The nurses say he slept like a baby last night."

After examining Father More, I agreed with Norman's evaluation. "Father, you're doing a lot better today."

"Thank you, Doctor," he replied, smiling. "I feel almost as good as new. I must have a very good doctor."

And Mike Kennedy must have laid it on pretty thick last night, I thought to myself.

"When you've finished seeing your other patients, I would appreciate a few minutes of your time," Father More continued pleasantly.

"All right, Father," I said, certain that he would again try to talk me into letting him leave the hospital early. "I'll come back after rounds."

I returned, resolved to be pleasant, but firm. From a medical point of view, there was no room for bargains or compromises. Father More's survival had been a matter of heartbeats, and I did not want him put in unnecessary jeopardy again.

"Would you mind if I called you Richard when we're alone? It's a lot more comfortable than Doctor. Frankly, except for Mike Kennedy, I've never cared much for doctors. You can call me John."

"That's fine with me. What's on your mind?"

"Carole told me I had a cardiac arrest yesterday. The experience was rather strange. It felt like I was floating above my body looking down at myself and everyone."

"You mentioned something about that yesterday."

Father More's eyes drifted toward the ceiling. "I felt as though I was bathed in this white light. It was so peaceful. Then something released, and I awoke on the gurney." Father More paused. "Last night, I was returned there. It was as if I'd spent my life in darkness, and had been lifted up and cleansed by a beautiful healing light." Father More turned his gaze toward me.

"They could have been magical dreams of some sort, I suppose, but they seemed so vivid and real. I'd like to know what you think, from a medical point of view."

I was astonished, not only by what Father More was telling me, but by the change that had come over him. The priest seemed so vulnerable and human.

"Other patients have described experiences similar to yours during a cardiac arrest. They're called near-death experiences. Several theories, from medical to metaphysical, have attempted to explain them, but I don't think anyone really understands what they are, or what they mean."

Father More ignored my answer. "I've understood since childhood that God sent His son, Jesus, to earth for mankind's salvation, and that Christ was crucified for our sins. Would you like to know why I'm so certain?"

I nodded.

"Because I am the embodiment of sin." Closing his eyes, Father More grimaced. "God knows how wicked I've been, and why my father had to discipline me so severely. He was a hard man. Made my life hell."

A surge of sympathy welled up in me for this tortured soul. "I'm sure you weren't nearly as bad as all that, Father."

Father More's face hardened into a dark scowl. "I was a contemptible bag of excrement."

"Father, I think you should know that Mike Kennedy mentioned some of the things your father did to you when you were a child."

"Yes, Michael told me. My father was trying to teach me discipline and strength of character. They were important lessons."

"Lessons? For what it's worth, I think beating you like that was a criminal act. You must have felt enormous anger toward your father. I know I would have. It would have been perfectly natural."

Father More winced. "He'd close the door to my room and remove that big black belt ever so slowly, while ordering me to bend my naked backside over the chair. He wasn't satisfied until my bottom was raw and blistered. Then, he'd begin on the backs of my thighs and legs, whipping me until I buckled under the pain, all the while shouting at me to stand up and be a man. I'd try to hold on, swallowing the pain and straining not to cry, while my mother banged on the door, sobbing hysterically. She was always too terrified to do anything, except for that one time."

"When was that?" I asked.

"Once, during a particularly vicious beating, my mother opened the door and threw herself into the room. She got down on her knees between us, put her hands together and pleaded with him to stop before he killed me.

"My father kicked her in the stomach, and screamed at her to get out. She rolled into a fetal position, whimpering like a dog while he kept kicking her in the back, then in the head. Somehow my mother managed to crawl out of the room. He slammed the door and grabbed the belt, panting and sweating like a rabid dog. That's when it came over me."

"What happened?"

"I turned and faced him. All fear left me. I looked straight into his eyes, and said, 'I want you to die. I am going to pray for you to die every day.'

"My father's face turned purple. He whipped me across the face, and I reeled across the room, fell over the chair, and went down. By now, my father was so out of control that nothing could stop him. He went berserk and began whipping and kicking me until the pain stopped. Everything became numb, and I lost consciousness.

"From that day until the day he died, I prayed for my father's death." Father More's eyes grew dark. "So you see, I learned about the power of prayer as a small boy. I learned that my prayers could kill."

"You thought you were responsible for your father's death?"

Father More looked at me evenly, and continued without a trace of emotion. "At my father's funeral, everything was very orderly. Our parish priest read his eulogy about what a wonderful, god-fearing man my father was, while my mother sat weeping, and the uniformed policemen from his precinct stood in perfect formation.

"I stood alone at the far side of my father's gravesite, staring at the casket, holding my breath, and waiting for the priest to stop the eulogy and point his finger at me. I knew it was just a matter of time before he announced what I had done, and the police would take me off to some hideous hell where I would spend the rest of my wretched existence being beaten and tortured.

"Then, a miracle happened. As they lowered my father's casket into the ground, I heard the voice of Jesus. I stepped back and glanced around, but I was alone. The Lord spoke again, clearly and distinctly: 'You who have sinned must surrender your soul to me.'

"I whispered to Him, 'How can you forgive me for what I've done, dear Jesus?' He answered, 'Devote your life to my glory, and you shall receive salvation.' From that moment on, Christ became my savior.

"Of course, the weight of the cross has not always been easy to bear. God's word is strict and demanding. But I would have borne anything to save my soul from eternal damnation." Father More looked at me. "Do you believe man has an eternal soul?"

"As a physician, I've always been more preoccupied with life in the here and now than with immortality, Father."

"Of course. Life is to be revered because life is God-given. As a doctor, you should know that better than most."

"To be honest, most doctors these days view the human body more as a machine than a God-given wonder. It may sound coldly scientific, but from a pragmatic standpoint, the approach usually works. My experiences have taught me that people are a lot more than the sum of their bodily parts. Guess I'm a little old school."

"I'm a little old-fashioned myself," Father More said, smiling. "What are your beliefs about the hereafter? About sin and salvation?"

"I don't know much about those things, Father. My patients seem more ridden with fear than sin."

Father More's eyes narrowed to steel slits. "Well, you should. No matter how weak and frightened a man might be, his main order of business is to save his soul."

∞

After leaving Father More, I headed to the nurses' station, where Carole intercepted me. Unfolding an electrocardiogram strip, she said, "At 3:15 this morning, Father More had a new episode of ST elevation on his EKG. Look at this." Carole pointed to the alarming strip. "At the same time, his blood pressure bottomed out. Went down to 60 over 40. The episode only lasted a minute or so, but there was another recurrence at about four o'clock."

The new ST segment abnormalities on Father More's electrocardiogram were alarming. It suggested that another coronary artery might have become unstable. In all likelihood, a fresh clot on the second vessel momentarily occluded it. Fortunately, the clot had failed to attach itself long enough to cause heart muscle damage, but the cumulative effect on Father More's heart function resulting from the momentary occlusion had been disastrous. A blood pressure of 60 over 40 could not sustain life.

While focusing on the disturbing implications of Carole's discovery, I also found myself wondering if the episode coincided with Father More's strange experiences. When his blood pressure fell to 60 over 40, Father

More's brain would have been temporarily deprived of oxygen just as it had been during the cardiac arrest. Whatever had triggered his out-of-body experience during the arrest could have been responsible for its return last night.

The urgency in Carole's voice snapped me out of my reverie. "Something is happening. Father More is not stable!"

"What do you suggest, Carole? Aren't we doing everything we can right now?"

"Yes, but I'm terrified."

"Me too. At this point, I suppose all we can do is wait, and hope."

Late that afternoon, my secretary buzzed the intercom. "Carole just called. You'd better get up to the unit. Father More's in trouble."

Grabbing my lab coat, I raced up the three flights of stairs to the coronary care unit.

Norman, Carole, and the medical team were all milling about in Father More's room. I motioned Norman out of the room to tell me what happened.

"The priest's having another coronary. He's in severe chest pain, and there are big-time new abnormalities on the electrocardiogram."

"What about his vital signs?"

"We're getting a weak blood pressure, but it's only 60 over 40, and dropping. Father More's in major-league shock. He needs the counterpulsation balloon."

A quick assessment confirmed Norman's evaluation. The electrocardiogram showed that ST segment abnormalities were now present on nine of the twelve EKG electrodes, an unequivocal increase from the original six. A new portion of the heart had been damaged, and the cumulative effect on our patient's heart and blood pressure was catastrophic.

"Father," I said, moments after we had given him intravenous morphine to lessen the pain, "you've had another heart attack, and your blood pressure's quite low. We need to use a medical device that will assist your heart. It's temporary, and after a few days, your heart should recover sufficiently to work on its own."

Despite being semiconscious, Father More seemed to understand that he was in serious danger. Looking up, he mumbled, "Whatever you think, Doctor."

Once we threaded the device near the priest's heart through an artery in his groin, and had the balloon working, our patient's blood pressure immediately improved. But I was far from reassured. The device had stabilized him for the moment, but we had been forced into a grim race against time. All of us knew that our patient's fate now depended on whether his heart would heal before the inevitable side effects of the balloon were unleashed.

Carole shook her head as she came out of Father More's room.

"Come on now, Carole," I said, "let's stay optimistic. Father More is going to make it."

I felt myself becoming tense and irritable—a sure sign of the anxiety I always felt when one of my patients was in trouble.

"Well, he's okay for now," Norman said, "but what if we can't wean him off the balloon? How are we going to decide when to call it quits? After all, we only have a few days, and the man is a priest."

Again, my apprehension about this possibility showed itself. "We'll cross that bridge when we come to it," I snapped. "And, damn it, I don't think we'll have to make that decision."

I looked at Carole. She turned away.

In the days that followed, a disquieting pattern developed. Father More remained stable while on the counterpulsation balloon, but each time we attempted to wean him from the device, his blood pressure plummeted. And with each passing day, his blood pressure slowly drifted downward, even when the balloon was working at full capacity.

At the same time, something unusual began to take place. Father More was not in shock or a coma, and he responded lucidly whenever he was asked a question, but his eyes remained closed. The priest's body was as motionless as an Egyptian mummy, and seemed oblivious to the endless cacophony of doctors, nurses, and technicians bustling and babbling amid the myriad machines and monitors surrounding him. As the days went on, his disconcerting stillness appeared to deepen.

On the morning of day five, we entered Father More's room and were startled to discover that our patient had opened his eyes, and looked quite alert. "How am I doing, Doctor?" he asked, looking directly at me.

"Okay, Father," I said, lowering my eyes to avoid his.

"You haven't made any progress getting me off the balloon, have you?" Reluctantly, I shook my head.

"How much longer do I have?"

"Oh, we still have plenty of time," I lied, but my tone betrayed the wretched reality imposed by the indifferent ticking of fate's clock. I wanted to be honest with Father More, but I did not want to extinguish hope—his hope or mine.

"I'm still optimistic," I said into the pall that enveloped the room. "Are you in any pain? We can give you something…"

Father More shook his head. "Medication will not relieve my pain."

"What do you mean?"

"My life has been a lie. I've spent it preaching that Jesus punishes us for our sins, that man is conceived in sin, and that we must repent or be condemned to hell for all eternity. I've had so little to say to the tortured souls that came to me seeking solace in God's love, about forgiveness and mercy."

"Father, I'm sure you've given great comfort to…" But before I could continue, Father More turned away.

∞

"What did you make of *that*?" Norman asked, as we walked down the hall. "Father More's out of it for days, and suddenly he wakes up, and out comes all this remorse. It's kind of bizarre, don't you think? To be honest, I don't know what's keeping the man alive. For the last twenty-four hours, his blood pressure has been hovering close to 75 despite the balloon, the IVs, the meds, everything. He should be in shock by now."

"I think Father More knows he's dying, and it's compelled him to confront his life. I can't imagine anything worse than having to confront death and discovering that you're repulsed by the way you've lived. It must be especially painful for a religious person who's been devoted to doing what he thought was God's work. As for his not going into shock, I can't answer that one. What do you make of all this, Carole?"

"Earlier this morning, Father told me about some of the experiences he's been having."

"What kind of experiences?" Norman asked.

"He's been seeing…he's been having visions."

"Visions?" Norman said. "What kind of gobbledygook is that, Carole? What's going on with Father More happens all the time to patients who aren't getting enough oxygen to their brain. In case you haven't heard, they're called hallucinations."

Shaking her head as if she was about to address an insolent child, Carole said, "Tell me, Doctor, does anyone really know what a so-called 'hallucination' is? Isn't hallucination another fancy medical term you doctors made up so you can put a label on something you know nothing about? It allows you to hide behind impressive-sounding jargon without having to admit to anybody—including yourselves—that you're clueless."

"Au contraire, Carole. I will now explain the word *hallucination* to you," Norman said, feigning great sagacity. "A hallucination is when somebody's seeing things, and hearing things that ain't there, okay? Ain't enough oxygen going to the brain. Comprende?" Norman was on a roll, and grateful for the respite, I sat back, enjoying their banter.

"The old nervous system gets out of whack and goes haywire. Brain chemistry's all screwed up. Nerves going crazy, firing out of control. Hallucinations are about messed-up brain chemistry and crazed nerves. They got nothing to do with magical, mystical visions."

"Out of his mind is exactly where Father More is," Carole said, "and maybe someplace far beyond our understanding. You asked why Father hasn't gone into shock and died. Maybe he's been clinging to life to try to make peace with God. You're a good doctor, Norman, but you've got a lot to learn."

"Okay, gang," I interrupted. "Let's cool it. This nightmare has all our nerve endings a little crazy."

∞

At five o'clock the next morning, time ran out.

Norman called me with the news at home. "I'm afraid Father More's spiked a high fever, and his blood is hemolyzing."

Hemolyzing meant that the balloon had now begun to destroy Father More's red blood cells.

"Any luck weaning him off the balloon?"

"Zero. And to make matters worse, even with the thing at full tilt, his blood pressure is dropping. What are we going to do?"

"Start a slow drip of intravenous norepinephrine to stabilize the pressure. I'm coming in."

Father More's eyes were closed when we entered the room. "Father," I said. "Can you hear me?" A faint smile crossed his lips.

I looked at the monitor. The blood pressure was dangerously low, hovering around 55 over 40, and the balloon was barely helping. "Let's change the balloon synchronization and see if we can get it to… "

"Already tried that," Norman said.

"Well, we're going to try it again."

After I unsuccessfully reworked the balloon, Carole pulled me aside. "The temp is up to 105," she said. "The hemolysis has made him jaundiced, and his red blood count is way down. Father is severely anemic."

Jaundice is a condition caused by an excess of a chemical called bilirubin in the bloodstream that seeps into the skin and eyes, turning them yellow. In Father More's case, bilirubin was accumulating because the balloon was destroying his red blood cells, and they were now pouring the substance into the bloodstream. In turn, the rapidly decreasing red blood cells spurred the anemia.

"Maybe the fever is being caused by an infection," I said. "Let's get blood cultures, and start him on antibiotics. We'll treat the anemia with blood transfusions to keep pace with the red blood cell destruction. Order two units of fresh red cells."

"Let's face it," Norman said. "Father doesn't have a functioning heart left. Even if we find an infection, you know we aren't going to get anywhere. Even with the norepinephrine drip, his pressure's starting to drop again."

"Then increase the drip, Norman."

"Okay," he said, moving toward the nurses' station muttering under his breath. "But it's not going to work, and you know it."

Of course, Norman was right, but I felt compelled to try *something*. Anything. Feeling helpless and not knowing what else to do, I returned to my patient's bedside.

At the foot of Father More's bed, I reached out and touched his frozen, pulseless feet. His exposed legs were mottled with the baseball-size blotches of broken, bleeding blood vessels. Under the sheets, his bony body seemed to be melting away. But while Father More's withered frame lay cold and lifeless, his face, freed of its fearful furrows, emitted a golden glow. Was it the effect of the jaundice? Or could there be something more?

"John, it's Richard," I said.

"Come closer," Father More said in a hoarse whisper.

Sitting down on the side of the bed, I leaned toward him.

"A miracle has happened. The Lord has answered my prayers." Father More paused to catch his breath.

"All I've ever wanted was to know Him. Now, He has graced me, and I am at peace." My patient laid an icy hand on mine. "I'm ready to go."

∞

After John received last rites, Carole waved me into the room for a final farewell. A clean white sheet covered Father More's body. The lights had been lowered, and in the shadows behind his bed, the flashing signals on the now mute monitor screens flickered as faintly as candles. In the faint light, Father More's face looked luminous.

Silently, I took his hand in mine. Father More's eyes remained closed as his crusted lips began to move.

"I'm in the light—so radiant." Father More's hand weakly squeezed mine. "It's... I'm home." His hand went limp.

Father More was gone.

Unable to let go of my patient's hand, I stared at his lifeless face, mesmerized by its golden glow. Time passed—how much I do not know.

Then, there was a hand on my shoulder. It was Carole. Gently, she led me out of Father More's room.

∞

After calling Mike Kennedy, who graciously thanked me on behalf of Father More's parish for our efforts, I turned to Carole.

"What do you think, Carole?"

"John allowed us a glimpse into the great mystery. A hint that there's more than we can ever know."

"I think so too."

∞

Years passed before I could begin to comprehend the gift that Father More had given us. Only in retrospect did it become clear that he had opened a door through which Norman, Carole, and I entered, forever changing our lives.

While retaining the veneer of his New York personality, Norman became a quieter, more reflective person. He also became religious, attending synagogue regularly, and steadfastly observing his Jewish faith.

Carole supplemented her clinical skills by learning to use alternative healing techniques to unblock and release energies that augment health. She also developed a seminar program on death and dying for health care professionals.

∞

Father More's confrontation with death opened me to possibilities that were nonexistent in the scientific and intellectual traditions in which I had been raised. Over time, I began to explore realities that transcend those we know through science and technology. As the physicist Werner Heisenberg wrote, "Scientific concepts cover only a very limited part of reality, and the part that has not yet been understood is infinite."

Medical science teaches that we are biological beings, functioning according to physiological principles that are governed by genetic codes and their biochemical elaborations. Father More showed me that such reductionist notions are simplistic, and don't begin to recognize or value the vast complexity of human beings. William James said, "Rational consciousness as we call it, is but one special type of consciousness, whilst all around it, parted from it by the filmiest of screens, there lie potential forms of consciousness entirely different....No account of the universe in its totality can be final which leaves these disregarded....They cannot furnish formulas. They open a region, though they fail to give a map."

All of us have experienced moments when we are lost in a sunset, the rapture of love, or a religious experience. At such times, the ordinary sense of our separateness evaporates, and we often feel at one with the universe. Perhaps in those moments, we have briefly entered another reality not dissimilar to what Father More described during his out-of-body experiences.

Were Father More's experiences hallucinations—abnormalities of brain chemistry and nerve function caused by oxygen deprivation? Or were they visions—vivid, life-altering occurrences during which something appears within one's consciousness that profoundly affects the heart and soul, perhaps even under the influence of a divine or spiritual dimension?

What I do know is that Father More's experiences altered my consciousness. When I sat holding his hand as he died, I sensed an unmistakable presence. Normally, watching one of my patients die devastates me. But at the moment of Father More's death, I was filled with wonder. I too felt released from ordinary reality, and was witness to a profoundly spiritual process. Losing a patient for whom I cared deeply no longer tormented me. Everything about Father More's passing seemed right, even holy. In that moment, my own state was so blissful that it frightened me. The foundation of my everyday being had fallen away, and I too was perfectly at peace. As inexplicable as it was, nothing has ever seemed more real.

Father More's most powerful teaching was about death—our greatest fear. He allowed me to see that death may not be an end, but a possible path to other realities. Human consciousness has been called spirit or soul—the part of us that religions throughout history have referred to as eternal. The animating energy that is consciousness—something medical science cannot locate in the anatomy of our physical bodies—might, at the moment of death, simply change to another form within the miracle of existence.

Einstein wrote: "I feel myself so much a part of all life that I am not in the least concerned with the beginning or the end of the concrete existence of any particular person in this unending stream." I have continued to employ the technology of modern medicine in the treatment of my patients, but there has been a change. Before my experience with Father More, I regarded the death of a patient as a defeat. I no longer believe that. Instead, I have come to put more trust in the ultimate outcome. I fight for life, while allowing for death.

Paradoxically, accepting death with more equanimity has enriched my reverence for life. Both are mysteries beyond human reason. I have been with many patients at the moment of their death. Father More graced my life by allowing me to glimpse beyond, and to appreciate the miracle of existence as an exquisite mosaic about which we can only wonder. A realm we can only name—perhaps, like Father More, by calling it God.

Glossary

Adrenaline. A secretion of the adrenal glands (also called epinephrine) that constricts blood vessels, and increases heart rate and blood pressure.

Aneurysm. A saclike bulging of the heart or a blood vessel due to weakening by disease, trauma, or a birth defect.

Angina pectoris. The symptoms of discomfort (pain, tightness, squeezing, or other sensations) resulting from a decrease in blood supply to an area of the heart muscle.

Angiogram. An X-ray examination of the heart or blood vessels after a dye is injected into the structure to be studied.

Angioplasty. A catheterization technique in which a balloon or other device (such as a laser) is used to widen the opening of an obstructed artery.

Antianginal. A drug or other treatment that relieves the symptoms of angina pectoris.

Antiarrhythmic. A drug or other treatment that controls or prevents heart rhythm disturbances.

Anticoagulant. A drug that inhibits blood clotting, and enlargement of preexisting clots.

Antihypertensive. A drug that lowers blood pressure.

Aorta. The largest artery of the body, originating from the heart and transporting blood to smaller arteries that supply the body.

Aortic valve. The structure between the left ventricular chamber of the heart and the aorta.

Arrhythmia. A disturbance of the heart rhythm.

Arteriosclerosis. Hardening of the arteries. A broad term applying to various conditions that cause the walls of arteries to thicken and lose their elasticity.

Atherosclerosis. A type of arteriosclerosis in which the wall of an artery is infiltrated by cholesterol and other materials. When these deposits enlarge, they project into the inner portion of the artery and obstruct the flow of blood.

Atrial fibrillation. A chaotic heart rhythm affecting the two upper cardiac chambers.

Atrium. One of the two upper cardiac chambers.

Auscultation. The act of listening to the heart, lungs, and other parts of the body with a stethoscope.

Blood thinner. An anticoagulant. Medication that decreases the ability of blood to form clots.

Bruit. A sound heard with a stethoscope over a blood vessel caused by blood turbulence. Its presence may indicate the presence of an obstruction.

Cardiac. Pertaining to the heart.

Cardiac arrest. The cessation of heart pumping activity, usually caused by a chaotic heart rhythm called ventricular fibrillation.

Cardiac catheterization. The insertion of a thin tube into a vein or artery and its advancement to the heart to study its function or take x-ray pictures called angiograms.

Cardiovascular. Pertaining to the heart and blood vessels.

Cardioversion. The restoration of a normal heart rhythm by means of an electrical shock applied across the chest.

Carotid arteries. The two blood vessels that provide blood to the right and left sides of the brain.

Catheter. A thin tube of plastic or other material.

Cerebrovascular accident. A stroke. Partial or total paralysis of a portion of the body due to brain malfunction caused by a decrease in its blood supply.

Coagulation. The formation of a clot.

Coma. A state of prolonged unconsciousness from which a patient cannot be aroused.

Coronary artery. A blood vessel on the surface of the heart that supplies a portion of it with oxygen and nutrients.

Coronary thrombosis. The formation of a clot on the inner surface of a damaged coronary artery lining. The term is often used to refer to a heart attack.

Deep vein thrombosis. Blood clots in the leg veins.

Dilatation. The enlargement, widening, or opening up of a portion of the heart or a blood vessel.

Diuretic. A drug that increases the amount of salt and water excreted by the kidneys.

Dysautonomia. A nervous system imbalance resulting in an excessive response to stress.

Dyspnea. Difficult or labored breathing.

Edema. A swelling due to an inflammation, or to an accumulation of salt and water in the body.

EEG. An electroencephalogram. A test measuring the electrical activity of the brain.

Ejection fraction. The fraction of blood that is ejected from the heart with each beat.

Embolism. A blood clot fragment that has broken off from a larger clot, traveled in the bloodstream, and lodged in a vessel elsewhere in the body.

Emphysema. A pathological accumulation of air in the tissues of the lungs, most commonly the result of pulmonary damage caused by smoking.

Epinephrine. A secretion of the adrenal glands, or a medication that constricts blood vessels and increases the heart rate and blood pressure.

Extrasystole. A premature heartbeat.

Femoral artery. The main artery supplying blood to one of the legs.

Fibrillation. A chaotic heart rhythm that causes the heart muscle it affects to cease effective contractions. Atrial fibrillation involves the upper atrial chambers, and causes a twenty- to thirty-percent decrease in the output of blood from the heart. Ventricular fibrillation involves the lower ventricular chambers, and causes cardiac arrest: cessation of all cardiac function.

Fibrinolytic. Having the ability to dissolve a blood clot.

Gallop. A sound heard over the heart, indicating heart dysfunction.

Heart attack. The death of a portion of the heart, usually caused by an occlusion of one of the coronary arteries.

Heart failure. The condition brought about when cardiac function weakens to the point where it becomes incapable of pumping sufficient blood to meet the needs of the body.

Heart-lung machine. An apparatus that provides oxygen to blood diverted from the heart during open-heart surgery.

Hemolysis. The destruction of circulating red blood cells.

Heparin. An anticoagulant that prevents blood from clotting and already existing clots from enlarging or breaking off.

Hypercholesterolemia. Excess cholesterol in the blood.

Hypertension. High blood pressure.

Hypertrophy. An increase in the mass of heart muscle.

Hypotension. Low blood pressure.

Hypoxia. Low oxygen level in the blood.

Intra-aortic balloon counterpulsation pump. A catheter threaded into the aorta with a balloon on its tip that rhythmically expands and deflates to improve heart function.

Ischemia. A temporary imbalance between the oxygen needs of a portion of the heart muscle and the oxygen supply provided by one or more obstructed coronary arteries.

Jaundice. A condition caused by an excess of bilirubin in the bloodstream that seeps into the skin and eyes, giving them a yellow appearance.

Kerley B lines. Linear streaks on a chest x-ray that indicate the presence of fluid in the lungs.

Lasix. A diuretic drug that increases the amount of salt and water excreted by the kidneys.

Lipid. Fat.

Lipoprotein. A compound consisting of fat and protein that carries fats such as cholesterol through the bloodstream.

Lumen. The channel inside a blood vessel.

Mitral valve prolapse. A condition in which a variation in the size, shape, or structure of the mitral valve causes one or both of its leaflets to balloon or billow into the left atrium when the left ventricular chamber contracts.

Murmur. A sound that can be heard with a stethoscope over the heart or an artery, caused by turbulence of blood flow. Murmurs can be innocent (of no significance) or can indicate an abnormality, as of a heart valve.

Myocardial infarction. Damage of an area of heart muscle due to inadequate blood supply. A heart attack.

Myocarditis. An inflammation of the heart muscle, most commonly due to excess alcohol intake or a virus.

Myocardium. The heart muscle.

Open-heart surgery. An operation on the opened heart, during which blood is diverted through a heart-lung machine.

Panic attack. The appearance of sudden, overwhelming fear, with or without cause, that produces hysterical or irrational behavior.

Pathogenesis. The origin of a disease.

Percussion. A method of detecting disease by tapping the fingers over the lungs or other parts of the body.

Pericarditis. An inflammation of the pericardium, the sac surrounding the heart.

Phlebitis. An inflammation in a vein (often in the legs), accompanied by a blood clot.

Plaque. A buildup of cholesterol and other fatty and cellular deposits in the wall of an artery.

Plasma. The liquid portion of the blood with the blood elements removed.

Pneumonia. An infection or other inflammation of the lungs.

Prognosis. A prediction of the future outcome of a disease or other medical condition.

Prophylaxis. Preventive treatment.

Psychosomatic. Referring to a disorder caused by the mind and emotions, characterized by symptoms that mimic those of a disease.

Pulmonary edema. A severe form of heart failure, or other condition, in which substantial amounts of fluid collect in the lungs, causing severe shortness of breath.

Pulmonary embolism. The lodging of a blood clot or other fragment in a pulmonary artery after breaking off from another clot, usually located in the legs.

Pulmonary. Pertaining to the lungs.

Rales. Abnormal crackling or rattling sounds heard over the chest, caused by disease of the lungs.

Respirator. A machine that delivers oxygen-rich air to the lungs, usually through a breathing tube inserted in a patient's windpipe (trachea).

Rheumatic heart disease. A cardiac condition caused by damage to one or more of the heart valves.

Saturated fat. A fat that cannot absorb hydrogen. A diet high in these fats can cause high blood cholesterol levels.

Sclerosis. A hardening.

Septicemia. An invasion of bacteria into the bloodstream.

Shock. A state caused by a failing circulation, characterized by low blood pressure; low urine output; cold, clammy skin; and a decrease in mental acuity.

Stenosis. The narrowing of a heart valve or artery.

Stethoscope. An instrument for listening to the heart, lungs, and other organs in the body.

Stroke. A partial or total paralysis of a portion of the body caused by brain damage, usually due to vascular disease.

Syncope. A faint.

Syndrome. A set of symptoms due to a common cause.

Tachycardia. A rapid heart rate.

Thrombolytic. Ability to dissolve clots; such an agent.

Thrombophlebitis. Inflammation and clot formation in a vein, usually in the legs.

Thrombosis. The formation, development, or presence of a blood clot.

Vascular. Pertaining to blood vessels.

Ventricles. One of the two lower cardiac chambers. The right ventricle pumps blood to the lungs. The left ventricle pumps blood through the aortic valve to the aorta and the rest of the body.

Ventricular fibrillation. A completely chaotic heart rhythm that causes cardiac arrest.

Ventricular premature beats. An early beat or contraction originating in the ventricles.

About the Author

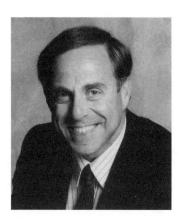

Richard Helfant is a Harvard-trained cardiologist who pioneered the development of cardiac electrophysiology and nuclear cardiology. He was founder and Medical Director of the Philadelphia Heart Institute, one of the first facilities in the U.S. to use balloon angioplasty and calcium channel-blocking drugs.

Dr. Helfant's positions include Professor of Clinical Medicine at the University of Pennsylvania School of Medicine, Chair of the Department of Cardiology at Cedars-Sinai Medical Center in Los Angeles, Professor of Medicine at the UCLA School of Medicine, and Vice-Chair and Professor of Clinical Medicine at the UC Irvine School of Medicine.

Widely published in the medical and scientific fields, Helfant has written more than 200 scientific articles, editorials, and book chapters, and three textbooks for physicians. He is also the author of *Women, Take Heart*.

Dr. Helfant lives in the Los Angeles area. For more information, see his website, *richardhelfantmd.org*.

Sentient Publications, LLC publishes books on cultural creativity, experimental education, transformative spirituality, holistic health, new science, and ecology, approached from an integral viewpoint. Our authors are intensely interested in exploring the nature of life from fresh perspectives, addressing life's great questions, and fostering the full expression of the human potential. Sentient Publications' books arise from the spirit of inquiry and the richness of the inherent dialogue between writer and reader.

We are very interested in hearing from our readers. To direct suggestions or comments to us, or to be added to our mailing list, please contact:

SENTIENT PUBLICATIONS, LLC
1113 Spruce Street
Boulder, CO 80302
303.443.2188
contact@sentientpublications.com
www.sentientpublications.com